HEALTH CARE
HALF-TRUTHS:
TOO MANY MYTHS,
NOT ENOUGH REALITY

HEALTH CARE HALF-TRUTHS: TOO MANY MYTHS, NOT ENOUGH REALITY

ARTHUR GARSON JR., MD, MPH, AND
CAROLYN L. ENGELHARD, MPA

ROWMAN & LITTLEFIELD PUBLISHERS, INC.
Lanham • Boulder • New York • Toronto • Plymouth, UK

ROWMAN & LITTLEFIELD PUBLISHERS, INC.

Published in the United States of America
by Rowman & Littlefield Publishers, Inc.
A wholly owned subsidary of The Rowman & Littlefield Publishing Group, Inc.
4501 Forbes Boulevard, Suite 200, Lanham, Maryland 20706
www.rowmanlittlefield.com

Estover Road
Plymouth PL6 7PY
United Kingdom

British Library Cataloguing in Publication Information Available

Library of Congress Cataloging-in-Publication Data

  Health care half-truths : too many myths, not enough reality / Arthur Garson Jr. and
Carolyn L. Engelhard.
     p. ; cm.
  1. Medicine—Miscellanea. 2. Medical care—Miscellanea. 3. Social medicine—
Miscellanea. 4. Health care reform—Miscellanea. I. Engelhard, Carolyn L., 1951–
II. Title.
  [DNLM: 1. Delivery of Health Care—organization & administration—
United States. 2. Health Care Reform—United States. W 84 AA1 G1755c 2007]
R708.G18 2007
  610—dc22   2006034330

  ISBN-13: 978-0-7425-5829-8 (cloth : alk. paper)
  ISBN-10: 0-7425-5829-0 (cloth : alk. paper)
  ISBN-13: 978-0-7425-5830-4 (pbk. : alk. paper)
  ISBN-10: 0-7425-5830-4 (pbk. : alk. paper)
  eISBN-13: 978-0-7425-6591-3
  eISBN-10: 0-7425-6591-2

Printed in the United States of America

⊗™ The paper used in this publication meets the minimum requirements of
American National Standard for Information Sciences—Permanence of Paper for
Printed Library Materials, ANSI/NISO Z39.48-1992.

To our children Lauren, Kathleen, and Caitlin.
You will get it right; you already have.

While all men are entitled to their own opinions,
they are not entitled to their own facts.

—Daniel Patrick Moynihan

CONTENTS

PART III   QUALITY: THE MYTHS OF GOOD CARE

PART IV   COVERAGE: THE MYTHS OF INSURANCE, UNDERINSURANCE, AND UNINSURANCE

PART V   THE FUTURE

ACKNOWLEDGMENTS

The idea for this book came during "health care reform" of the 1990s when one particularly prominent public person made a claim about reform that wasn't completely untrue—but mostly untrue—and was published across the country as gospel. This then became the first myth. We would like to express our appreciation to that person for getting us started in attempting to bring reality to the myths. We would also like to thank Mike and Trina Johns, who honed the myths; our wonderfully bright students who challenged the myths and sharpened our thinking; Jenny Minott, our research assistant, who did so much more than just pull references and chase down statistics; Shirley Rothlisberger, who, with the greatest of cheer, kept us on track from the original draft to the final sendoff; Don Fry, who helped to make our sentences declarative and our ideas clearer; and most importantly, our spouses, Suzan and Vic, who kept us sane—or as good as it gets.

INTRODUCTION

Aren't you tired of hearing that the American health care "system" is broken? Well, it is: your bill that can't be understood—or paid; your eight-minute doctor visit; your own child who was just laid off, and whose family has no health insurance. Our health care system will not be fixed by those in back rooms; each of us, in our own way, will have to work on it—whether directly as practitioners or indirectly as voters—or our health will continue to get worse.

This book informs Americans about American health care, ways in which it is tarnished and ways in which it shines. We must begin with a common set of information; our current information comes from sound bites that on their surface seem perfectly reasonable, but on closer examination are wrong.

In these pages we will deal with the most common of these myths, beginning with the two whoppers about the U.S. in comparison with the world.

PART I—OUR COUNTRY AND THE WORLD

Chapter 1

MYTH: American medical care is second-rate compared with other countries.

REALITY: The life expectancy for an African American man in Harlem is lower than the life expectancy in Bangladesh. Because of murders, drug abuse, and forty-six million uninsured, our life expectancy ranks twenty-third in the world. Life expectancy is an index of the HEALTH of our population; only ten percent of health is contributed to by MEDICAL care—which is what doctors do—such as coronary bypass surgery. While it is not ideal, medical care in the United States is among the best in the world: you don't see people getting on a plane to go to Europe for better medical care. America is always getting picked on for being the most expensive with "nothing to show for it." We *are* buying expensive medical care, but actually have plenty to show for it. Don't confuse health care and medical care: there is a world of difference.

Chapter 2

MYTH: American health care is the most expensive in the world.
REALITY: Our spending per person *is* the highest in the world—we spend almost twice as much as number two Switzerland; the costs are higher largely because we insist on doing everything for everybody with the latest and greatest technology and drugs, our administrative costs are absurd, we add profit into virtually every transaction, and our prices are much higher in the U.S. than other countries for drugs, doctors, and hospitals. But read the myth and remember what we said above: these statistics are actually MEDICAL CARE costs; we have no idea what our HEALTH CARE costs, because we would have to include programs that affect health, such as expensive social programs for education, welfare, and the prison system. That's not how countries usually compare themselves; if they did, we might not look so bad.

PART II—COST: EXPENSIVE CARE

Chapter 3

MYTH: America wastes one-half of its medical care dollars.
REALITY: We really do waste a lot: on doing too many procedures (e.g., taking prostates out) and giving out medicines that are not always needed

(e.g., antibiotics for colds); we spend huge amounts of money on diseases that people bring on themselves because they are obese or they smoke; we waste money on outdated administrative systems in which electronic procedures could save a lot; we pay doctors for every single service, which creates bad incentives to do more; we sue and sue, upping the cost of insurance for doctors and the amount of care. We do waste a lot but we probably don't waste half of our dollars. Why does this matter? Even if we cut waste by as little as five percent we could pay for the uninsured.

Chapter 4

MYTH: Most medical care dollars are spent in the last six months of life.
REALITY: We spend a lot—actually it is ten percent—in the entire last year of life. But fixing that is another thing: for starters, we don't know when that last year is going to start—no flag goes up and says, "You have a year left." Even when a patient and family are told, "there's a ninety-five percent chance you won't make it," they are sure they are in the five percent who will. Taking measures like giving "do not resuscitate" orders or providing hospice and advance directives generally will save money, but only about three percent because these decisions are made so late.

Chapter 5

MYTH: Better quality saves money.
REALITY: Certainly, we need to save money and keep medical care costs down—this is important for all of us. It makes sense that if we do the right thing, people would be healthier and that would save money. Right? The problem is that more often than not, doing the right thing turns out to be more expensive. For instance, how about taking drugs the way they are prescribed? Only one-third of patients on Medicare take the statin drugs (that reduce cholesterol) as prescribed; if all patients took their statin medication appropriately, it would cost Medicare approximately $10 billion *more* per year. *Not* taking these drugs may result in heart attacks, but the heart attacks that occur don't cost $10 billion. It turns out that only about half of Americans get "high quality" medical care—but most get LESS than they should, not more. And fixing the problem would cost more, not less.

Chapter 6

MYTH: Preventive care saves money.
REALITY: The cold truth is that screening the entire population for high blood pressure and treating huge numbers of patients with drugs for their entire lives is very expensive. Even assuming the treatment prevents strokes and heart attacks, the patient lives just long enough to get another expensive disease that can't be prevented, like pancreatic cancer. Sure, some preventive care can save money: measles vaccination, water fluoridation, and asthma inhalers for children, but most do not. Nonetheless, preventive care is a MUST. The purpose of health care is to be healthy, and prevention is effective in keeping us healthy. Just don't look for real money from savings on prevention that we can spend on other programs such as covering the uninsured.

Chapter 7

MYTH: America will not ration health care.
REALITY: America rations health care right now: We have forty-six million uninsured who die earlier because they do not have appropriate care. We ration by making it extremely difficult to sign up for public programs, such as the requirement to complete the sixteen-page application for Medicare drug benefits or the sixteen-page application for Medicaid that must be renewed every six months in person. Will we ever directly ration by restricting treatment that is known to be beneficial because the country can't afford it? America will hate it, but it will happen. We can't all have it all.

PART III—QUALITY: GOOD CARE

Chapter 8

MYTH: Science drives most medical decisions.
REALITY: You would like to think that doctors agree on what to do for a given patient, and that the treatment for a heart attack is the same in Boston as it is in Miami—but not so. In different parts of the country, the number of operations such as removing the prostate can vary by five to ten times. How can this be? A big part of the reason is that less than ten percent of medical care is based on the gold standard of science in patient care called

the "randomized clinical trial." You might not think this is so important, but trials provide unexpected answers: in one randomized clinical trial that looked at which commonly prescribed drug was best for preventing sudden death the results showed that ALL the treatment drugs in fact had MORE deaths than the sugar pill. In truth, most of the care we receive is based on a combination of data and opinion—some passed down from generations of teachers because their teachers said so. This is getting better, but for major decisions, asking for the basis of the recommendation and getting input from more than one physician is a good idea.

Chapter 9

MYTH: High quality care cannot be defined.
REALITY: Of course you can define high quality care. High quality care: (1) maintains and improves health; (2) doesn't waste money or other resources; (3) is safe—meaning avoids medical errors; (4) occurs when the patient needs it; (5) is responsive to the wishes of the patient; and (6) eliminates disparities in care by factors such as race, gender, and age. But despite the fact that we can define it, you should not assume you are getting it. All too often we assume the physician and hospital are top-notch. Learn to use quality "report cards" and pay attention to them.

Chapter 10

MYTH: Consumers can make the best decisions about their medical care.
REALITY: Consumers don't make great decisions about buying a car or car insurance, and in the same way they are not likely to make any better decisions about their health care. Most will say to doctors "fix me," just like they say to the mechanic "fix my car." For those that want to know about their health care (probably not as many as we would like to think), the materials that are available tend not to be presented in the way most patients or consumers find useful. The system will eventually change this and tailor the information to make it more useful for each consumer, but even so, there remains a real question about how many will use these materials in their decision making. Cost is pretty important; and the neighbor and sister-in-law are powerful advisors.

Chapter 11

MYTH: Fewer doctors will be needed as medicine changes.

REALITY: Can you get in to see any doctor you want this week? Of course not. There is a shortage of doctors today and it is going to get worse, not better. The Baby Boomers are going to create more demand by living longer and demanding care NOW; there will be fewer available physicians as women and men demand more time at home with their families and physicians decide to retire early. How about all that technology? New technology is going to take more new doctors to work it; we *will* be healthier, but doctors will still be needed to monitor our health and care for us when we get sick; and we will get sick. Electronic health records will certainly improve the quality of care, but at best they will save fifteen percent of a physician's time, maybe then doctors will be able to spend ten minutes with a patient instead of the current eight minutes.

Chapter 12

MYTH: The current malpractice system helps patients.

REALITY: There are close to 100,000 medical errors that cause death in the U.S. each year, the same as if a 747 jet crashed each day. For example, every day two patients either have the wrong limb amputated or the wrong kidney taken out. Most of these do not result in lawsuits; conversely, most lawsuits are not about actual medical errors—and most of the time, the injured patient is not compensated. Malpractice suits do not reduce medical errors; errors are prevented by physicians, nurses, and hospitals changing the way systems work in order to prevent mistakes before they happen. Even simple changes such as requiring the patient and doctor to mark the correct side of the body before surgery can reduce errors. Ultimately, it is the responsibility of the medical profession to admit mistakes, compensate patients for the errors that happen, weed out the bad apples, and make malpractice suits unnecessary.

Chapter 13

MYTH: Managing care is evil.

REALITY: There is nothing wrong with "managing care" that is defined as trying to promote the highest quality care for the most people and providing it efficiently. However, "managed care" was the Darth Vader of the 1990s and came to be viewed as having the primary goal of saving money by limiting choice of physician and by limiting access to good medical care. The Health Maintenance Organization (which really didn't maintain anything, or keep people healthier and was often not well organized) was Darth Vader's spaceship and it crashed and burned.

PART IV—COVERAGE: INSURANCE, UNDERINSURANCE, AND UNINSURANCE

Chapter 14

MYTH: In America, there is a "safety net" of government programs providing health care for the poor.
REALITY: Everybody thinks Medicaid provides health coverage for the poor. If it did, we wouldn't have forty-six million people without health insurance. No matter how poor you are, if you are between nineteen and sixty-four years old, for all practical purposes, you are not covered for health care in the United States. There are rare exceptions, such as being completely disabled, blind, pregnant, or having end-stage kidney disease. States do have some flexibility to help out parents whose kids are covered by Medicaid, but the parents essentially have to be not working. And, no matter what, there is no health coverage for adults without children. Period. More than one in five Americans will be uninsured by 2012. Why should you care? You could be one of them.

Chapter 15

MYTH: People who work can afford health insurance.
REALITY: Seventy-five percent of the uninsured are in a family that works. These are the people you know: the waiter, the clerk at the cleaners, or the cashier at the fast food place. Most work in small businesses and many small businesses do not offer insurance. Even if the business offered insurance, the premiums would be thirty to fifty percent of the entire family's income for a couple working at minimum wage. Buying health insurance becomes a luxury when you have to eat.

Chapter 16

MYTH: Provision of health insurance for employees has always been the employer's responsibility, and will continue that way.

REALITY: No rational policy group sat down and decided that employers should provide health insurance. This was actually a historical accident that started during World War II when, because they couldn't increase wages, businesses were permitted to give certain employee benefits (e.g., health care coverage) instead of salary increases, and the benefit was tax-deductible to the employer. It stuck for a while. Now, it is becoming un-stuck: less than sixty percent of all businesses are offering health insurance (down from sixty-nine percent five years ago), and small businesses aren't the only ones being affected—look at General Motors.

Chapter 17

MYTH: The uninsured get the care they need in emergency rooms.

REALITY: Emergency departments are for emergencies; they are not set up for preventive and follow-up care. But the uninsured do get most of their care there because they have nowhere else to go. Even so, overall, the uninsured get about half the medical care as the insured. No wonder they have a twenty-five percent higher death rate.

Chapter 18

MYTH: No additional funding is needed to cover the uninsured; the money is available in the system.

REALITY: Covering the uninsured would cost approximately $83 billion per year more than we currently spend on medical care in this country. This money is in the system: possibilities include cutting waste in medical care or reducing administrative cost, or eliminating the tax deduction for employer-based insurance or even rolling back the recent tax cuts, but everyone has an excuse for why that won't work. The money is there, it's just not available.

PART V—THE FUTURE

Chapter 19

MYTH: All other developed countries provide health care coverage for everyone; we should be no different.
REALITY: The reason that we do not have a Canadian health care system is that we are not Canadian. We are uniquely American: we are rugged individuals, entrepreneurial (not only health care manufacturers, but also physicians and lawyers); we fear government control; we need simple sound-bite messages; we want white teeth; we are swayed by powerful interest groups; and we swing from liberal to conservative every thirty to fifty years. Any health care system, in order to succeed, must recognize and address these factors and catch the wave at the right time. So far, it hasn't happened.

Chapter 20

MYTH: Major change in the American health care system is impossible.
REALITY: When St. Peter was asked whether the United States would ever have a rational health care system, he answered, "Not in my lifetime!" But we disagree: it WILL happen, and yes, we will tell you in this chapter briefly what we really think should happen and how—so read on.

In this book, we provide the facts so that each of you can fit the pieces together, take part in the decision-making process, and propose better solutions.

We wanted the book to be an "easy read" and so chapters 1–20 are uninterrupted by reference numbers. But, to paraphrase Moynihan (in the introductory quote), we are accountable for all the facts in the book. The sources for the facts, as well as suggestions for further reading, chapter by chapter, make up the last half of the book.

Enjoy.

I

OUR COUNTRY AND THE WORLD

❶

MYTH: AMERICAN MEDICAL CARE IS SECOND-RATE COMPARED WITH OTHER COUNTRIES

HEALTH CARE AND MEDICAL CARE ARE NOT THE SAME THING

Although we hear lots of complaints about how bad the U.S. health care system is, how often do people go to other countries for their hip replacement or heart surgery? Not very often. That is because surgery and medical treatment is medical care: what doctors, other health practitioners, and hospitals do. In fact, our MEDICAL care *is* among the best in the world. For example, in the United States, death after a heart attack has declined seventy-five percent over the last fifty years, and middle-aged Americans today can expect to live three to five years longer than they did in 1950 as a result of medical treatments for heart disease. If we look at how our medical system serves sick Americans, we do quite well. On the other hand, infant mortality and life expectancy, which describe HEALTH care, *are* second rate and place the United States in the bottom quarter of industrialized countries.

Does the distinction between health and medical care make a difference? You bet it does. Maintaining health includes not only medical care but also a large number of socioeconomic and environmental factors, such as poverty and lack of health insurance. Therefore, the ways of improving health care versus medical care are also very different. Although medical care and health care can improve, the health care system is truly broken in this country. We have to attack the problems with fixes that are largely *not* medical care: Did you know that the life expectancy for an African American male in Harlem is lower than the life expectancy in Bangladesh? All the medical care in the world will not fix that.

HEALTH CARE

Life Expectancy

Life expectancy is the average number of years men or women are expected to live from the time they are born. It is often used to gauge a country's overall health. At the beginning of the twentieth century, life expectancy in the United States at birth was forty-seven years. The overall life expectancy is now about seventy-seven years, and based on age-specific death rates, individuals aged sixty-five years can expect to live on average another seventeen years or so, a dramatic improvement over the last 100 years. Yet, despite these improvements in life expectancy in the United States, we rank only twenty-third among developed countries. How can this be in a nation that prides itself on medical innovation and quality of life? The answer lies in the multiple factors that determine the "health" of the people in a nation, and therefore their life expectancy.

What Affects Health?

First of all, gross domestic product, socioeconomic status, level of education, and occupation greatly influence health. In the United States, there are highly significant disparities in health care related to race, ethnicity, education, socioeconomic status, and living in either rural or inner-city areas. For example, the life expectancy at birth for an African American man is sixty-eight years, seven years less than for a white man in 1990, with the gap narrowing to less than six years by 2002. African Americans are more likely than any other racial or ethnic group to develop cancer, and thirty percent more likely to die from it. Inequalities in income and education underlie many of the disparities in health and are related: the death rate for people with twelve years or less of education is more than two and a half times the rate for persons with thirteen or more years of education, and lower income and education levels are associated with higher levels of violent crime and more deaths due to firearms, motor vehicle accidents, and substance abuse. Higher incomes permit increased access to medical care and allow people to afford better housing and live in safer neighborhoods. Have you ever thought about the fact that many people who live in slums don't have an address? As a result, they may not be counted at the time of a national census, and they certainly do not receive notification of benefits that could be related to education or health care, such as schools and Medicaid. In addition to racial and ethnic disparities in health, life expectancy is also tied to social status. Race and social status are both associated with the health of individuals, although it is often difficult to separate the two. No matter how rich or poor a country is, there is a "social gradient" in health and disease: in Europe and the United States, one's occupation, income, and education have all been shown to predict mortality. Those with higher social positions at the top of the socioeconomic scale have better health than those at the bottom. Perhaps it is because those at the "bottom" have less control over their environment and more stress, which is associated with increased risk of heart disease, absence from work, mental illness, and earlier death.

Second, certain behaviors and environmental factors contribute to the health of our population. Smoking, alcohol consumption, and obesity are all related to life expectancy, and the physical environment can bring harm to individuals as well as communities. High environmental pollution in inner cities caused by automobile exhaust is associated with asthma, chronic bronchitis, heart disease, and lung cancer. In fact, individual behavior and environmental factors are responsible for a significant percent of all premature deaths in the United States. On the other end of the spectrum, good environments improve individual and community health: with more physical activity, better transportation options, and urban planning. Cities that have green space for walking and opportunities for social interaction as part of community living are related to longer life expectancy, particularly in the elderly.

Third, whether one can get access to medical care clearly influences life expectancy. Being able to see a doctor or other practitioner is often related to what type of health insurance one has. These "tickets" to the medical system—health coverage through insurance and access to timely care—will be discussed later in chapters 14 through 16. It is sufficient here to point out that there is a strong relationship between health insurance and life expectancy. Lack of health insurance compromises people's health because they are less likely to receive preventive care and more likely to be diagnosed in the late stages of disease, which results in loss of productivity and costly hospitalizations. Just having emergency rooms, public hospitals, and community health centers that provide a medical "safety net" is not enough: having insurance alone improves overall health and reduces mortality rates by as much as ten to fifteen percent.

The last determinant of life expectancy is medical care, which includes what is done by physicians and hospitals, and is measured to a large extent by the outcomes of illnesses, as well as the likelihood of staying healthy. Despite the importance of medical care in diagnosing and treating disease, it has been estimated to delay premature death only about ten to fifteen percent of the time. Therefore, improvements in the quality of medical care alone will have a limited impact in reducing early deaths over the whole population.

Being serious about improving health means going beyond expanding medical care; we need to change unhealthy behaviors and improve the environment as well. As we end our discussion of life expectancy, it is worthwhile to point out that the World Health Organization just added another category: "Deaths Due to Terrorism." Clearly, terrorism has little to do with medical care and a lot to do with larger social factors, and illustrates why life expectancy is more an index of health care than medical care.

Infant Mortality

Infant mortality is the percent of infants dying in the first year of life. The United States infant mortality rate is twenty-seventh among developed countries, and twice the rate in England. Low birth weight and premature infants are responsible for the vast majority of infant mortality in the United States.

Let's get one important myth out of the way. Prenatal care does affect infant mortality and *is important*, but prenatal care—medical care—changes infant mortality much less than you might think because behaviors, lifestyles, and conditions such as smoking, substance abuse, and poor nutrition are also related to birth outcomes.

Low birth weight is the leading cause of death in the first month of life. The United States has the highest rate of teen pregnancies in the developed world, and we know that younger mothers have more premature babies with low birth weight. But we also know that cigarette smoking and alcohol are factors for low birth weight. In addition, higher infant mortality occurs in inner cities and among the uninsured. However, when we adjust or eliminate the effects of all of those factors, race is still the dominant factor in infant mortality. In the United States, the African American infant mortality rate is two and a half times higher than the rate among white, Hispanic, and Asian infants, and has not changed in thirty years. Racial and ethnic differences in infant mortality are found throughout the developed world and add to other factors, such as smoking and age of the mother. It is important to continue to pursue long-term answers as to how we might decrease the infant mortality rate in the United States, but our best near-term approaches are likely to be social and behavioral. Lowering teenage pregnancy rates, along with reducing maternal smoking, drug and alcohol abuse, and poor nutrition will go a long way toward improving the health of mothers and newborns. Not only will lowering teenage pregnancy rates improve infant mortality, it will also improve life expectancy; remember, the death of an infant counts in life expectancy.

MEDICAL CARE

Medical care is best defined as what practitioners *do*. Physicians and other medical professionals certainly take care of the sick. Increasingly, we will also be held accountable for keeping people well: not only for counseling about prevention, but also for the percentage of our patients who stop smoking and avoid obesity.

Medical care can be described by a number of outcome indicators (in other words, "what happens") such as survival rates for patients with diseases like cancer, kidney or liver transplant, or heart attack. Outcome indicators can also be calculated for preventable problems, such as how many patients have hepatitis B, whooping cough, and measles, or even how many children die from childhood asthma. In recent studies comparing medical care indicators in the United States, Canada, England, Australia, and New Zealand, the United States does quite well in the area of clinical effectiveness. None of the five countries scores consistently the best or worst overall, and each could improve the quality of care for its citizens. In the United States, for example, breast and prostate cancer survival rates were higher than in other countries, but U.S. survival after kidney or liver transplant is lower than the other countries. This may in part be because of differences in patient characteristics since the United States, unlike other countries, routinely offers organ transplants to older patients and to those whose first transplant has failed. And, the U.S. system has shorter or no waits: just five percent of Americans wait longer than four months for an elective surgical procedure compared to a quarter of Australians, Canadians, or Britons. Interestingly, Australia ranks seventh and Canada ninth in life expectancy (way ahead of the United States), and yet when we look at outcomes of medical care, including survival rates after the age of sixty-five, the U.S. performs about as well as other countries. However, this does not mean that we cannot improve our medical care; recent studies point out how, despite our history of effective and innovative medical treatments, our system of medical care can perform better.

In summary, the United States is a complex blend of different cultures. That's what makes us great and strong. While it is tempting to "adjust" for infant mortality or life expectancy because of socioeconomic status or the crime rate in Harlem, we are what we are. We should not excuse or explain away our health care problems, but begin to attack them through improvement in our social and public health systems. We can most definitely improve our medical care as well, but improving medical care may prove to be the easier task.

MYTH: AMERICAN HEALTH CARE IS THE MOST EXPENSIVE IN THE WORLD

WHAT COSTS ARE WE MEASURING?

In the United States we haven't a clue what our real health care expenditures are, but the rest of the world doesn't know what they spend, either. We have just seen in Chapter 1 that there are important differences between what is considered health care and medical care. Health care is broad and includes social factors such as poverty. Medical care is only part of health care, as it is largely made up of what happens between patients and doctors, such as mortality from a brain tumor. We spend a lot on medical care, but the distinction between the two is important. If we don't realize the larger scope of health care, we might conclude that our medical care system is responsible for an individual's overall health, when medical care is a very small part of the picture, as we pointed out in Chapter 1.

Similarly, we have difficulty trying to measure how much money we spend on health care vs. medical care. To calculate health care expenditures, we would need to include widespread social expenses, such as law enforcement to combat violent crime, a portion of prison costs as a deterrent to crime, the cost of city green space construction to permit jogging, a portion of the cost of after-school programs to help deter teen pregnancy, a portion of welfare payments to combat poverty, subsidized housing, and costs borne by children of the elderly who care for their parents at home, to name a few.

IS THE UNITED STATES SO DIFFERENT FROM OTHER COUNTRIES?

The comparative statistic across countries is called National Health Expenditures (NHE). "National Medical Care Expenditures" is a more appropriate term since NHE typically measures spending on medical care rather than on the larger activities that influence health care. In 2004, the NHE (we're stuck with the term) for the United States totaled almost $1.8 trillion. For each dollar, thirty-one cents purchased hospital care, twenty-two cents paid physicians and other health care professionals, ten cents purchased prescription drugs, seven cents went toward nursing home care, and the remaining thirty cents was spent on other kinds of services such as program administration, home health care, and dental care. These are chiefly *medical care* expenditures.

So, the appropriate question to ask when comparing the United States with other countries' National Health Expenditures is whether our *medical* expenditures are the highest in the world. In fact, they are. We spend about fifteen percent of our gross domestic product (GDP) on medical care. But think for a moment about GDP: what does the percent of GDP have to do with anything? The gross domestic product of a country measures the total value of what the country produces. For example, every country, whether the United States, Canada, or those in sub-Saharan Africa, must have their GDP add to 100 percent. The differences in the categories that make up GDP, and the priorities each country gives certain services, points out how spending growth in one priority area might decrease the funds available for other services. For instance, what does it mean that Canada spends ten percent of its GDP on health care but only one percent of GDP on defense while we spend fifteen percent on health care and four percent on defense? One of the reasons why Canada can spend less on defense may be that it has a neighbor to the south that spends a lot on the defense of North America. On the other hand, Canada spends a greater percentage of its GDP on "social programs" compared with the United States. If you are homeless in Canada during the winter, you could freeze to death (no warm climate like Florida there), and therefore social programs become an even more important portion of overall "health care."

A more reasonable measure than GDP is health spending per capita, which tallies total health care spending divided by the number of people in a country. This figure shows how much countries spend per person. Even so, our per capita spending is the highest at $5,267; the closest European country behind us is Switzerland at $3,446 (about sixty-eight percent of the U.S.). The average for all other industrialized European countries is $2,193 (about forty-four percent of the U.S.). But, remember, these are *medical* care expenditures.

THE REASONS FOR HIGHER MEDICAL CARE SPENDING

Why is medical care spending higher in the United States? There are five main reasons:

The first reason has to do with the price of our medical care. Physicians in the United States are paid around three times more than physicians in other developed countries and hospital payments are also three times higher. Spending on pharmaceuticals in the United States is double that in Europe and Canada because the prices in the U.S. are higher, not necessarily because we use more drugs. In addition, many health-related industries in the United States, such as some insurance companies and some hospitals, are private, for-profit, and often traded publicly. Few other countries have for-profit organizational arrangements in health care, and most other industrialized countries distribute new technologies more slowly than we do, which slows health spending.

It is not the number of doctors, nurses, or hospitalization. Although some think the United States has the largest number of doctors, we actually have fewer physicians per 1,000 population than the European average (2.7 vs. 3.1), fewer nurses per 1,000 (8.1 vs. 9.0), and fewer hospital beds per 1,000 (2.9 vs. 3.9). Compared with France, our patients spend sixty-four percent of the time in the hospital (700 vs. 1,100 bed days per 1,000) and have fifty-three percent of the doctor visits (4.2 vs. 7.9 per person per year).

Second, in virtually all other countries, there is a single health care system that, with great bargaining power, sets prices for physicians, hospitals, and pharmaceuticals. Our mostly private system allows medical technology and new medicines to come to physicians and patients more quickly, and often they are used more often. However, for this privilege we pay the price—the Medicare Modernization Act of 2003 prohibits Medicare from bargaining with drug manufacturers, therefore preventing the large federal program to use its purchasing power to lower prices.

Third, the United States does not have a system of centralized medical decision making. Other industrialized countries weigh the costs of new technologies along with the benefits, which slows the introduction of new medicines and treatments. Most Americans would not support this model for use in the United States for fear that new medical advances would be delayed, but the centralized medical decision-making systems in other countries do reduce spending. For example, in England, the government simply does not pay for certain drugs that are very expensive and thought to be "of little benefit." However, this lack of centralized decision making leads to fragmentation because of the variety of private and public insurance plans and various payment systems. In the United States, providers are rewarded for doing more, not less. Compared with single-payer systems such as Canada, health services in the U.S. are more expensive, patients are treated more intensely, and hospitals are less efficient.

The fourth reason the United States has higher costs than other countries is because of our administrative complexity. Overall administrative costs in the United States have been estimated at twenty-four percent of health spending, almost one in every four dollars. Let's take the example of a single patient who comes to the clinic. A billing clerk must determine whether the patient has insurance, which may require a telephone call to the insurance company (and time is money when we are put on "hold"). The physician sees the patient and orders a number of tests. The insurance company will have rules about which tests are covered, and either the physician's office or the laboratory doing the tests will need to check on whether the tests require "pre-approval" by the insurance company. "Pre-approval" means that the insurance company needs to tell the practitioner whether, for example, the insurance company will pay for a particular type of x-ray. Continuing our example, the patient is also given several prescriptions; the pharmacy then goes through a similar process to determine which drugs are covered by the insurance company and for how much. After seeing the physician, having tests, and picking up the prescription, the patient begins receiving bills. Many of the bills cannot be understood, and patients do not pay because they do not understand, again, at a "cost" to the system since the bill is issued yet another time, and ultimately turned over to a collection agency if the bill is not reconciled. Consider this set of procedures and compare it with any other country's health system without our collection of multiple payers, each with their own forms to fill out, pre-approval and coverage rules, and complex billing.

The final reason can be explained by our relative wealth as a country. The gross domestic product per capita has a direct bearing on how much health and medical care we consume. Not surprisingly, those countries with higher earnings and greater spending have people who request more health care. Clearly, the ability to pay for medical care will have an effect on the amount one consumes, and so it is no surprise that the United States has a larger appetite for medical care. If America's gross domestic product per capita was the same as Switzerland's, the difference between our two countries' health care spending per person would be much smaller—only eighteen percent more instead of the reported forty-four percent.

Medical malpractice is a commonly cited reason for higher U.S. health spending, and politicians, physicians, and the media all call for a reform of the medical malpractice system in the name of controlling health care costs. Capping malpractice awards has been on the legislative agenda in Congress and in most state houses, and most physicians will admit to practicing expensive "defensive medicine" to avoid being sued by their patients. However, despite the fact that malpractice litigation is a problem in the United States, as well as in other countries, there is little evidence that it is a serious component of health spending in the U.S., making up less than one percent of total health spending. And although it is possible that practicing defensive medicine contributes more to health spending than the costs of medical malpractice, experts report an upper estimate of nine percent of health spending is likely attributable to defensive medicine.

There is widespread agreement that the United States spends too much for medical care per capita, and that if we changed some of the ways we paid for health care, integrated the administrative and clinical systems of care, and eliminated some of the bureaucracy, it would be less expensive.

For example, if administrative costs went from approximately thirty percent to five percent (found in other systems around the world and in our own Medicare system), we would still spend more than most developed countries but be more in line with higher income nations such as Switzerland. Is it possible for the United States to bring our health costs more in line with other countries and save money? This is the topic for Chapter 3.

II

COST: THE MYTHS OF EXPENSIVE CARE

(3)

MYTH: AMERICA WASTES ONE-HALF OF ITS MEDICAL CARE DOLLARS

America wastes one-half of its medical care dollars? Where did *that* number come from? It came from a landmark study in 2002 that reported that in some regions Medicare pays more than twice as much per person as it pays in other regions with little or nothing to show in health benefit for the increased spending. We do waste a lot of dollars on medical care, but this "one-half" estimate is based on an over-zealous interpretation of the data; the number is more likely one-third. And whether the waste is one-third or one-half, consider this: if we (only) wasted five percent of the $1.8 trillion we currently spend in our medical care system ($90 billion) and, if we could capture this five percent, we could, for example, provide medical care coverage for all of the uninsured.

TOO MUCH MEDICAL CARE

The data supporting the claim of wasting one-third of our dollars come from studies that point out important differences in how we practice medicine, examining how often we do procedures (such as prostate surgery and coronary bypass surgery) or how well we care for patients with chronic illness (like diabetes and heart disease) for Medicare enrollees in different parts of the United States. Physicians in one part of the country may do a procedure as much as three to ten times more frequently as those in another part of the country *with the same eventual results* in terms of longer life or better quality of life. Some areas of the United States, such as Boston and Miami, spend far more than others, such as Minneapolis, even when similar patients are matched to be sure that there are not sicker patients in one part of the country than another. When these data are then applied to the entire Medicare population, and then ultimately the entire health care system, the logical conclusion is that if every doctor practiced in the same way as those do who provide the least number of procedures with the same overall results, we could (and presumably should) do thirty percent fewer procedures across the country, and then overall costs would decrease by thirty percent.

While the concept that we give too much care to patients could be sound, we should be careful about applying this reasoning to the entire system. The studies are based on specific procedures or for specific conditions in the elderly, and may not reflect overall medical care (for example, strokes, cancer, and heart attacks) in that population. The studies leave out those under the age of sixty-five, who are not covered by Medicare. Perhaps even more importantly, the studies were based on "looking back" at what happened to people after a decision was made either to do or not do a procedure. Beware of such conclusions; they are disturbingly similar to "what would have happened if I had bet on the right horse in the Kentucky Derby." We all work with the data we have at the time of the decision, "Should I have done those tests or not?" Clearly, as better data are becoming available about who needs which tests or procedures, these data are then available to the physicians and their patients as they make their decisions. And in some decisions, there is room for a difference of opinion (as we will see in Chapter 8).

We come to the conclusion that these studies looking at the use of procedures and chronic care services in the elderly point out a serious problem in our medical care system: patients are treated differently based on what state they live in, where they are treated, and how many practitioners there are in the region. As a result, we now have to look harder and smarter at better ways to identify what we should *not* be doing in our medical care system, and then not do it.

WHAT DO WE MEAN BY WASTE?

"Waste" is "doing things that provide no possible benefit to the patient." What sort of "things" do we mean? Clearly "rework"—repeating tests by one physician that another did yesterday—is a waste (sound familiar?). Another less obvious example is "Come back in three days, and let's check your ankle again, and get another x-ray." It will surprise you, but there are precious few data on how often patients need to be seen in "return visits," whether for acute care, such as an ear infection, or chronic disease, such as following a heart attack or hip replacement.

We also do not know whether an actual face-to-face visit is needed, or if a telephone call or e-mail might be just as effective. "Just as effective to whom?" you might wonder; *some* patients want to be seen in person, whereas for others, a phone call is enough, or may even be better because of convenience. Many times, only laboratory tests are needed, and a visit to a practitioner isn't necessary at all. However, at present, many patients seem to feel that when they come for lab tests, they must also visit the doctor. When a face-to-face visit is necessary, some patients insist on seeing a doctor, and others are perfectly comfortable seeing a nurse. Understanding patient preferences and appropriateness of practitioner may reduce waste, as well as new technologies that may streamline care. In 2001, about three million people sought advice for a specific medical condition online. In the future, as e-mail and tele-visit technology improves, and models for care involving integrated physician-nurse teams begin to appear, what patients and practitioners find to be "optimal interactions" may change, particularly for the ten percent of the population that uses seventy percent of health resources.

More and more, care will become even more of a partnership between the physician and patient. Patients will need to take increasing responsibility for the use of resources as they become better educated about when they need to be seen and when they don't, and when they need medicine and when they don't, rather than the current feeling by many patients, for example, that they or their children must receive antibiotics for viral upper respiratory infections. They will need to work with their physician and other health care team members to manage their chronic illnesses and practice positive preventive care by, for example, eating in a healthy way and stopping smoking. This is not always easy, because the current health insurance system rewards practitioners for doing more and because patients would often rather just take a pill than change their behavior. This combination often leads to using more services that are expensive and ultimately wasteful. High-quality shared decision-making requires patients to become informed partners who, with the help of their physician, better understand available treatment options and their consequences. Sometimes better treatment is actually doing less, and patients often have a difficult time choosing to do less—something we'll discuss in more depth in Chapter 10.

Another potential area of waste is the fear of malpractice. As we discussed in Chapter 2, you might ask whether practitioners see patients more frequently, order tests or even do procedures because they're worried about being sued. There is less of this day-to-day worrying by physicians than you might think or read about in the newspapers—but it is still there. Nonetheless, there is most definitely waste within the malpractice system, some—perhaps as much as nine percent of total health spending—may be ascribed to physicians practicing defensive medicine but some is dependent upon our court system and the way we determine who is at fault, and who gets paid. We discuss this problem fully in Chapter 12.

What else provides no value? How about administrative waste? After all, we spend more than $1,000 per person in the United States to administer our medical care system, compared with $307 per person in Canada. Reducing U.S. administrative costs to Canadian levels could save more than $300 billion annually. Doctors, hospitals, and insurance companies spend approximately eight to twelve percent on billing alone; compare that figure with the total administrative cost of our Medicare and Medicaid systems at three to five percent. It is likely that at least some of the inefficiencies in our system could be eliminated through the use of automated tools for billing, and we could significantly reduce costs.

The time practitioners spend face-to-face with a patient in an outpatient visit or in an inpatient hospital visit is about the same amount of time practitioners spend with the patient's medical chart. This should not be. Doctors waste time in providing extra documentation with lengthy notes in the medical record. Of course, it is important to document the visit, but why the extra work? One simple reason: to prove physicians are not committing fraud. The federal government and now private payers are insisting that hospitals and physicians document exhaustively in order to prove that they are not committing fraud. There are individual physicians (fortunately few) who bill for patients they have not seen, who see patients much too frequently, or who do more diagnostic tests than necessary in order to receive income from these tests. These physicians have caused increased awareness among the government and private payers. In what we believe to be an overstatement, the U.S. General Accountability Office has estimated that as much as ten percent of all Medicare and Medicaid billings are fraudulent. Moving toward a system that encourages and documents the use of best practices with the aid of electronic medical records may help move the emphasis away from fraud and abuse, and more toward demonstrating that the right things are done for the patient. For example, if the tests and treatments the patient receives are tied to national practice guidelines (and a difference from the guidelines is documented in the record) and billing is done automatically based upon what is documented in the chart, there would be less opportunity for mistakes in billing or outright fraud. Eliminating fraud would not only be the ethically correct thing to do in our medical system, but would also restore trust among practitioners, insurance companies, and the government. It would ultimately reduce the administrative costs of proving whether fraud did or did not occur.

ASSESSING "WASTE" IN MEDICAL CARE

Thus far, we have been assuming that waste in medical care is defined as "no benefit," which is very different from "a little benefit." Just how much lengthening of life, and at what cost, is considered "waste"? Is it even reasonable to ask about cost? One of the real geniuses in the field of analysis of how we provide medical care was John Eisenberg, who said, "to suggest that medical decision making can be divorced from consideration of cost denigrates the complexity of patient care . . . almost all clinicians would agree that, at some point, the extra money spent on tiny improvements in clinical outcomes is not worthwhile and represents inappropriate practice." David Eddy helps us further: "in a field filled with uncertainty and doubt, the difference between 'when in doubt, do it' and 'when in doubt, stop' could easily swing $100 billion a year."

In many business situations, it is possible to do a straightforward "cost-benefit" analysis in which one can calculate a simple ratio comparing the benefit of an action in dollars divided by the cost of that same action in dollars. As long as the benefit is greater than the cost, the project is worthwhile for the business. For example, if a builder decides that he can sell a house for $300,000 and the house costs him $250,000 to build, the cost-benefit ratio is 300,000 divided by 250,000. Clearly, the builder should go ahead with the house because the benefit is mathematically greater than the cost. Now, when we try that analysis with medicine, we run into a problem because when we try to put a dollar value on the "benefit," which is the improvement of health and/or lengthening of life, it is difficult to figure the value of the added years of life in dollars. Attempts to value human life in pure monetary terms have been unsuccessful (this is not to say that lawyers have not attempted to claim lost wages into the future for an individual who has been injured); as we know, value of life certainly extends beyond the value of lost wages.

Therefore, what are we to do? We use "added years of life" as a measure of "effectiveness" and place the added years of life in the lower part of the fraction (denominator) with the cost of achieving those added years of life in the upper part of the fraction (numerator). This calculation is called a "cost effectiveness analysis," and is the current best method to assess the value of medical care (what we call "getting bang for the buck"). For example, if having coronary bypass at a cost of $50,000 increases the average length of life by ten years, the cost part of the ratio would be $50,000, the "effectiveness" part of the ratio would be "ten life years," and the cost-effectiveness ratio would be $5,000 per saved life-year. This is a pretty good value when you consider that air bags in cars cost about $100,000 per saved life year. Lower numbers represent better value—i.e., $5,000 per life year is better than $100,000.

Therefore, it does seem worthwhile to at least ask the question of how we can compare cost-effectiveness across different types of treatments. In fact, when we look at the cost effectiveness of common procedures that are done every day, such as coronary bypass surgery or hysterectomy, the cost-effectiveness is less than $50,000 per life year. Please remember, this is not an implication that each year of life is worth $50,000, but only the ratio of the cost of the procedure to the effectiveness; this calculation helps us put things in the right order from most to least cost-effective. Even heart transplants and implantation of defibrillators (that "shock" you back to life when your heart stops pumping) are in the range of $75,000 per life year. However, procedures such as liver transplants that are in the range of $400,000 per life year are clearly less cost-effective. Is it possible to "draw the line" and say that on the basis of a cost-effectiveness calculation, one should do procedures and treatments with a cost effectiveness or "X" or below, and should *not* do treatments or procedures with a cost effectiveness of "above X"? Many European countries have a "cost per saved life" cut-off in their cost-effectiveness determinations for the introduction of new medical advances, typically between $30,000 and $50,000. American health insurance companies and the government demand services that reflect higher cost-effectiveness thresholds, perhaps as high as $100,000 per added year.

Our country has tried one experiment with using cost-effectiveness determinations and cutoffs for medical care. The state of Oregon ranked the medical services within its Medicaid program on the basis of cost-effectiveness from those that were absolutely life saving, such as providing surgery when the appendix was about to burst (an appendectomy), to those judged to provide less long-term benefit such as chemotherapy for very advanced metastatic cancer. Oregon officials then decided they would go down the list of medical services ranked by cost-effectiveness and "draw the line" between services that were covered or not based on the amount of available state money each year. However, their first attempt to make a list of ranked treatments based on cost-effectiveness failed because they soon realized that using cost-effectiveness alone would screen out important medical services that did not take into account patient preferences and quality of life. For example, certain procedures such as HIV testing for otherwise normal women about to give blood is not "cost-effective" by a formula—but would most definitely be considered important because of the fear of transferring the virus through a blood transfusion. Clearly, much more work needs to be done on the determination of how to measure medical benefit and then how to apply that to medical benefit funding decisions. Even with numeric rankings, deciding *not* to do certain procedures involves complex ethical, legal, and social issues, further discussed in Chapter 7.

In the meantime, do we waste money on medical care? Absolutely. We do too many procedures, probably see some patients too frequently (either because of the physician or the patient), spend too much on malpractice, administrative costs, and paperwork, and a small percentage of health practitioners commit fraud. How much money do we waste? A lot, but not one-half of medical care dollars.

4

MYTH: MOST MEDICAL CARE DOLLARS ARE SPENT IN THE LAST SIX MONTHS OF LIFE

For starters, about ten percent of our medical care dollars are spent in the last year of life, and although spending per patient increases as death approaches, we certainly do not spend most of our medical dollars in the last six months. And, despite dramatic changes in the U.S. health care system over the last four decades, these statistics regarding the economics of dying have remained constant. Interestingly, the Netherlands, a country known for its aggressive policies on health care, including assisted suicide and euthanasia, also spends about ten percent of their dollars in the last year of life.

The U.S. statistics are based on Medicare patients (most over sixty-five years of age), who account for about seventy percent of all deaths each year; five percent of all Medicare patients die per year and spend almost thirty percent of the Medicare budget ($295 billion in 2005). Medicare patients who die spend about six times more in their last year of life than those who do not, which, according to the federal Medicare program, comes to about $25,000 for each person who dies, compared with the almost $4,000 spent per year for those Medicare patients who do not die.

So, are we spending $21,000 per person "extra"? Not exactly. Let's address the obvious issue first: do we know a year in advance that someone is going to die? Rarely do we have that information, even in those older than sixty-five. A red flag does not go up. But, if we could find such an indicator, that might help us decide how much to spend.

Secondly, would we act differently even if we knew we had less than a year to live? Perhaps less than you think: for example, about half of the patients with AIDS and severe advanced symptoms say that they would nonetheless want to be admitted to an intensive care unit and have cardiopulmonary resuscitation (CPR) should their heart stop beating. Why? Probably because most people think, "I can beat the odds—I don't believe your statistics—they are not about me." The most telling example of this was the failure of the APACHE system, a scoring system that gave ninety-five percent odds that a patient would die in an intensive care unit. Once a patient received such a prediction, the intent was that the amount of care delivered would be reduced. But this reduction did not occur. Why? Many people have trouble facing the reality of death and many of the patients and their families wanted to believe that they were not in the ninety-five percent odds of a death, but that they were in the remaining five percent that would beat the odds.

In addition, just as with other kinds of health care, the use of end-of-life care varies by race, ethnicity, and socioeconomic factors. For example, African Americans use twenty-five percent less care in the three years before death than white persons, but eighteen percent more in the last year of life, mostly as a result of inpatient care. Lack of familiarity with the health care system, language barriers, and a tendency not to acknowledge pain or admit one is close to death create barriers for Mexican Americans. These types of differences by socioeconomic status disparities in end of life care are seen in other countries as well, where patients of lower socioeconomic status were more likely to die in the hospital or express distrust of the medical system.

Even knowing and accepting death, we don't save so many dollars, partially because medicine keeps coming up with more things to do at the end of life. Three ways have been proposed to decrease costs and at the same time "do the right thing for the patient":

1. *Advance Directives*. You would think that advance directives such as a "living will" would decrease costs. Current studies do not show much (if any) savings, somewhere in the neighborhood of zero to ten per-

cent. Why? In part it may be because only one in five Americans have completed living wills or it may be that by the time the family has decided that the living will applies, the end is indeed close (a few days), and there is not much savings. The situation with Terri Schiavo (who had been in a coma for several years) was clearly not the norm, but think about it this way: even in her case, there was disagreement among family members and the physicians who worked with each of them regarding the chances of recovery. Therefore, it is likely that even if Terri Schiavo had written a living will, the document would not have prevented the long-term costs since a number of family members thought she was not sick enough to apply the living will, and in those cases, family members can override an existing document.

2. *Hospice.* Hospice is used most often for patients with advanced cancer, but more and more those with heart, lung, and cognitive failures are using it as well. In a study looking at the effects of hospice care in which all costs were counted, expenditures were four percent higher overall among those in hospice enrollees than among those not in hospice. Hospice care has not been shown to save money, except in cancer patients, where it can provide savings of seven to seventeen percent among patients with aggressive cancers diagnosed in the last year of life. For others, particularly the oldest patients with non-specific conditions such as dementia, expenditures actually increase at the end of life for patients using hospice services because the lack of a clear prognosis often leads to the use of more intensive services until right before death.

3. *Withholding "Futile Care:" Do Not Resuscitate.* When a patient is thought by the family and physician to be "beyond hope," an order can be written in the chart not to attempt to bring the patient back if their heart stops; this is called a "do not resuscitate" or DNR order. When patients with and without DNR orders are analyzed, their end-of-life costs are the same. The reason appears to be that the DNR order is generally written at a time late in the patient's course of treatment when savings will be minimal. Beyond DNR, the definition of "futile care" becomes a matter of debate. In addition, it is not always cheaper to withhold care: for example, withholding expensive chemotherapy may be traded for the need for expensive hospitalizations due to the complications of cancer. Determining what "futile medical care" is

and when to withhold it raises an important point: even if the patients and families at the end of life refuse "life sustaining" intervention, the patient may not require less care but care of a different kind. Even if the chemotherapy is refused, the chronic medication and radiation for pain may be just as expensive. Therefore, despite a belief that the use of advance directives, hospice care, and reducing "futile care" can save our health system money, it has been estimated that only 3.3 percent of all health care spending and only six percent of Medicare expenditures could actually be saved by using such practices.

We can look at this potential savings in two ways: first, it is insignificant since national health expenditures increase more than three percent every year and this is a one-time savings of less than one year's increase. We believe the second way is more important: we must stop doing what we should not be doing. If we can find the $50 billion (three percent) in ways everyone agrees should be saved, by providing all patients near death with medical treatments and support that are appropriate but not "excessive," that money could be spent to improve the health of others or saved entirely.

We leave you with this disturbing thought about the last year of life. Remember that those over sixty-five years cost, on average, $25,000 in their last year. A premature infant born at less than twenty-five weeks (normal being forty weeks) weighing less than one pound costs on average $202,700 for the initial hospitalization alone. Although premature infants make up a small percentage of the total number of births each year, they constitute about fifty percent of total hospital spending on infant hospital stays. The most recent data show that up to fifty percent of infants born very prematurely have major disabilities including mental retardation, language delay, hearing loss, and visual disabilities. In this chapter we have been focusing on costs in the last year of life, but costs in the first year of life will likely receive similar scrutiny as our nation examines the long-term benefits and costs of medical care.

5

MYTH:
BETTER QUALITY SAVES MONEY

Americans should be able to count on receiving quality care when needed, even if it doesn't save money. The important thing is making sure we do not waste resources and that the medical care received is based on the best scientific evidence possible. But how do we know whether the health care we receive is effective and safe, and delivers benefits we need and value?

DOING THE RIGHT THINGS "RIGHT"

The Institute of Medicine (IOM) is a national body that brings in health experts to study problems in the U.S. health care system and issue reports with recommendations about how to improve the quality of medical care. In the last few years, IOM study groups have written a great deal about quality problems. The overall opinions of the studies is that our health care system suffers from many quality "gaps," particularly when it comes to treating chronic illness, using information technologies to prevent medical errors, and adopting strategies to improve patient satisfaction. According to the IOM reports, a quality health care framework in the U.S. would embrace six aims. First, health care would be *safe*, which means avoiding injuries to patients from the care that is intended to help them. Second, the care must be *effective*, which means beneficial and based on scientific knowledge. Third, health care should be *patient-centered* and thus respectful of patient preferences and values. Fourth, quality care ought to be *timely*, reducing waits and harmful delays. Avoiding waste and promoting *efficiency* is the fifth aim, and ensuring that quality health care does not vary and is available to all regardless of gender, ethnicity, geographic location, or socioeconomic and insurance status is the sixth aim of *equitable* care. A health care system that incorporated these six improvements would be safer, more reliable, more responsive to patients, and more technologically sophisticated to deliver preventive, acute, and chronic care services. Within such a system, health care practitioners would work together better, fewer resources would be wasted, and patients would experience improved health with less pain and suffering. Now *that* would be high quality care.

DELIVERING HIGH QUALITY CARE MAY BE EXPENSIVE

High quality care then, ultimately, is defined as care that improves overall health within a system that promotes health. Delivery of high quality care is the right thing to do. Sometimes delivering high quality care also saves money. For example, if we eliminate waste, we are eliminating services that provide no benefit and also eliminate those costs. On the other hand, delivering high quality care does not always save money. Think about one obvious case: less than one-half of older patients who are prescribed statin drugs to lower their cholesterol are still taking their drugs as prescribed six months later; the other half have stopped taking the drug. This country currently spends $10 billion per year on statins, and increasing the percent of patients actually taking the drug to three-quarters would mean a $5 billion increase for the cost of statin drugs. Although the cost savings found when fewer people had heart attacks would balance some of these additional costs, the savings would not be $5 billion. Clearly, taking a statin as prescribed (assuming the prescription is correct) is better quality of care, but it is also more expensive.

In a broader view, a recent study in a large number of patients looked at the use of medical care that either helped prevent or treat some of the leading causes of illness and death. The indicators of quality care were based on established national guidelines for screening, diagnosis, treatment, and follow-up care for thirty acute and chronic conditions. The percentage of patients with each condition who received "quality care" was then measured. Some of the thirty conditions, for example, included treatment for alcohol dependence (with an indicator of high quality care defined as "whether a physician referred a patient with alcohol dependence for treatment"); asthma (quality: "whether long acting drugs are prescribed"); suspected breast cancer ("appropriate follow up from mass felt on physical examination"); colorectal cancer ("screening for high risk patients starting at age forty"); heart failure ("ultrasound examination of the heart before treatment"); coronary artery disease ("counseling to stop smoking"); and diabetes ("diet and exercise counseling").

Overall, only fifty-five percent of patients received the recommended quality medical care and forty-five percent did not receive the proper medical care when indicated. Think back to your school days: in any course we took, fifty-five percent is an "F." Why did so few patients receive the appropriate care? As we will see in Chapter 8, the chain of doing the right thing for the patient is long and, unfortunately, complex. It begins with a group of practitioners, usually physicians, writing guidelines to inform other physicians of the best current medical care. Next, the physician taking care of the patient has to actually read the guidelines and remember them, and then she or he has to conclude that the recommended guideline applies to that specific patient. The appropriate test or prescription has to be ordered by the physician, and then finally, and perhaps most importantly, the patient has to follow instructions; to get the lab test, such as a colonoscopy, or to get the prescription filled and take the medication as prescribed for as long as recommended. Given this chain of events, it is no wonder that only fifty-five percent of care received by patients is considered "high quality." The physician, patient, family, and society need to work on producing high quality care together. From the physician's standpoint, the most important quality advance is likely to be the electronic medical record, where a patient's history is displayed and guidelines appropriate to each patient's care "pop up" as a reminder at the time of the patient's visit. For the patient, medical care quality is a little more complicated because it means different things depending on the individual's preferences and health condition—but it certainly involves personal responsibility in managing their own care and that of their family. We will discuss this further in Chapter 10.

So back to the original question: Does high quality care save money? In this study looking at the care received for thirty common health conditions, forty-six percent of participants received less than the appropriate level of "needed" care ("underuse"), whereas eleven percent received more than what was recommended or appropriate ("overuse"). If we do the math, almost four times as many people received less care than too much care. Therefore, it would follow, at least from this study, that delivering high quality care might actually require spending considerably more at every level of medical care—preventive, chronic, and acute—in order to do the right thing most of the time.

Let us end where we began: It may not be cheaper to deliver high quality medical care, but delivering high quality care is what we should do because it will improve patients' health and quality of life. The problem is that many people think that providing high quality health care requires just eliminating inefficiencies and waste in our health care system. Some innovations, like the use of electronic medical records, do hold the promise of increased benefits, higher quality health care, and cost savings. But, the truth is that in addition to streamlining what we already do, delivering high quality care will require doing even more in diagnosing, treating, and managing illness and disease in partnership with the patient, all within a better system using electronic tools that are costly to develop and implement. A popular notion has been that if we provide high quality care, we can then take the money saved and apply it to other important purposes such as covering the uninsured. Not likely.

6

MYTH:
PREVENTIVE CARE SAVES MONEY

PREVENTION IS EXPENSIVE

"Of course," you say, "prevention saves money!" Actually, most of the time, prevention does *not* save money. Willard Gayle put it best: "Preventive medicine drives up the ultimate cost of health care to society by enlarging the population of the elderly and infirmed. The child who would have died from tuberculoses will grow up to be a very expensive old man or woman." Think about it; it's true.

Even worse, unhealthy habits such as tobacco smoking may actually *save* money as people who smoke die earlier and use fewer health care dollars. "This doesn't make sense," you say, "Smokers are less healthy than nonsmokers." But, although smokers use up to forty percent more medical care while they are alive, the overall costs to society are four to seven percent less because smokers die earlier. And there is the contradiction: something "good," like quitting smoking leads to something "bad," like increasing medical care costs.

What is going on here? Just like the argument about quality in the last chapter, prevention is *absolutely* the right thing to do: it improves quality of life and increases our life span, but it doesn't always save money. The overall expense of prevention depends on the number of people being screened and treated, the cost of the disease being prevented, and the timeframe. In other words, early treatment of breast cancer in a fifty-year-old postpones the expense of dying from a brain tumor at seventy. The employer who covered her at fifty saves money, and Medicare who covered her at seventy spends money, and the overall system did not likely save money.

Let's look at high blood pressure, diabetes, and measles.

THE COSTS OF HIGH BLOOD PRESSURE TREATMENT

Consider the case of high blood pressure. Patients with high blood pressure have higher rates of stroke and coronary heart disease and lower life expectancy. In preventing high blood pressure, the costs involved include, first of all, screening the entire population, a very expensive undertaking. Then, we would need physician follow-up. Approximately forty-three million Americans are thought to have high blood pressure; twenty-three million are treated and only about half of them are controlled—a quarter of the total.

Once diagnosed, treating a patient with high blood pressure requires physician visits, lab tests, and medications. But there are other costs as well, such as inadequate blood pressure control, not complying with therapy, and lack of follow-up care. So, in evaluating the costs of treating high blood pressure we would have to add up the costs of general screening of the population, the treatment costs of those identified as having high blood pressure, as well as the costs of those who were hypertensive but who never knew it, and became ill as a result of their condition. In 1997, $30 billion was spent on treating hypertension, of which about a third ($7 billion) went for medications.

Here is an estimate of the savings produced by controlling blood pressure; of those with severe hypertension:

- Forty-four percent will *not* have a stroke;
- Twenty-one percent will *not* have a heart attack;
- Ten percent will *not* get kidney disease; and
- Five percent will *not* go blind.

The cost savings in treating high blood pressure depends on how high the blood pressure is and the risk of having a stroke or a heart attack, and overall, treatment appears to recover only about twenty-seven percent of the cost of the treatment. Therefore, as you can see, the cost of prevention is about three to four times the cost of the diseases caused by high blood pressure. But that's not all. In that period of time, patients will contract another disease, and it is likely that the disease they die from will be as expensive as the one prevented. So, from an economic standpoint, for the case of hypertension, prevention saved the cost of dying from diseases related to hypertension, but ultimately contributed to more costs over time: the cost of prevention of hypertension plus the cost of dying from a disease not related to hypertension.

But, you might say, what about the economic value of living longer? Shouldn't we save money because those extra years of increased health are productive? After all, that *is* what prevention and quality health care is all about, keeping people healthy longer. But, as in the case of preventing high blood pressure, the ten years one gains over those with high blood pressure are years that mostly occur when people are retired and are receiving social security and Medicare. Although a person is extremely important to their family as a grandparent and to life-long friends, there is little money going back into the system after retirement. This type of calculation weighing the economic benefits and costs of prevention to society seems very cynical, but it makes the point that we control diseases like hypertension to add years of life and to promote health, not to save money. In the future, as people remain healthier until right before death, then prevention will save the overall system money—but not now.

THE COSTS OF DIABETES TREATMENT

The total annual economic cost of diabetes in 2002 was estimated to be $132 billion ($92 billion in direct costs), and represented eleven percent of our country's health expenditures at that time. People with diabetes have medical expenditures 2.4 times higher than they would if they did not have the disease. Careful management of diabetes is likely to be cost saving in the short to medium term since prevention of hospitalizations for blood sugar that is too high or too low will clearly save money. Tight control of blood sugar in diabetics reduces complications from the disease by twelve percent and increases life expectancy. The direct effect of controlling diabetes means a drop in kidney and vision problems, fewer complications of diabetes such as limb amputations, and a reduction of more serious complications such as coronary heart disease and stroke, which occur at twice the rate in diabetics. For diabetics with coronary heart disease, yearly costs to treat a heart attack or stroke is $7,352 per person above treating diabetes alone, compared with $1,087 for preventive treatments that protect against the same events (treatment costs 6.8 times as much as prevention). Since cardiovascular disease is the most costly complication of diabetes, accounting for almost $18 billion of the $92 billion annual direct costs, the greatest cost savings would be achieved by preventing heart attack and stroke.

But remember, while prevention of serious or fatal complications of diabetes such as kidney failure and heart attack are clearly the right thing, they also can increase costs over time. Balancing the overall costs with the overall savings from reducing complications is important when discussing the economics of prevention. As in the example of hypertension, prevention of the costly complications of diabetes would produce a cost savings for those at highest risk of a heart attack, a stroke, blindness, or advanced kidney disease, but it may not save much for those who may have the disease but are at low risk for the complications.

If you prevent a disease that has large costs throughout life you will save money *for that disease*. However, the diabetic or hypertensive patient who saves the most from treating the disease early (before the complications set in), will have other costly medical conditions as they live longer, and may eventually die just as expensively later in life from some other disease as they would have without preventive care. This is not to say that we shouldn't invest in preventive treatments for patients with chronic conditions like diabetes or hypertension; these types of services do improve health, and preventing the complications of diabetes is *the right thing*, but may not save money overall.

MEASLES VACCINATION

Measles vaccination, on the other hand, can actually save money. The measles vaccine was licensed in 1963, and its effect was quick and dramatic:

in 1964, there were about 450,000 cases of measles; and within a year, the number had dropped by almost a half. By 1986, the number of measles cases was reduced almost ninety-nine percent. In all, from 1963 through 1982, fifty-two million cases of measles were prevented, 5,000 lives were saved, and more than 17,000 cases of mental retardation requiring long-term care were avoided, with a savings to the medical care system and to society at large of approximately $5 billion. This is clearly a case where spending money on prevention yields cost savings later—however, the cost saving was due to the avoidance of a complication that did not kill the patient, but was very expensive requiring long-term care.

IS THERE A BUSINESS CASE FOR PREVENTION? WHOSE DOLLARS?

From the perspective of *employers*, prevention saves money *as long as the patients stay fairly healthy while they are working or until the age of sixty-five*, when Medicare pays for the diseases that prevention delayed. For example, employers should certainly pay for mammograms, since paying for advanced breast cancer is significantly more expensive.

How many times have you heard an argument like this: The employer doesn't want to pay for prevention because it is unlikely that the person will be working there long enough to see the benefits of the prevention. Why should I worry about the cholesterol if the prevention of the heart attack will be ten years from now, and my employee will be working for someone else?" At first glance there is not a strong "business case" for prevention, but there could be if one enlarges the business case to encompass all businesses together instead of as individual companies. After all, cardiovascular disease alone costs $142.5 billion a year in lost productivity. If the worker's previous employer had worried about his cholesterol for the last ten years, you would benefit, as the employee would probably use less medical care after you hired him. Extend this argument even further: as our country continues to move toward consolidation of major insurance companies, over time, there may be only a handful of health insurance companies in the United States covering virtually all people who have employer-based coverage. No matter who the employer is, the insurers would clearly see that it would be to everyone's benefit to cover prevention since they, as well as the patients and employers, will all eventually benefit in terms of staying healthier and having decreased absenteeism. So, prevention does save money for the employer as long as the employee is working because that particular worker, as well as all workers, stays healthier and more productive. In fact, each $1.00 invested in worksite health programs such as blood pressure control and medical self-management for acute illness brought savings of $3.48 in reduced health care costs and $5.82 in lower absenteeism costs. This is why the savings offsets the costs of prevention for those workers that remain productive as a result of maintaining their health.

The big picture, however, remains the same. From the standpoint of the expense to the entire medical care system from cradle to grave, prevention does not save money except in certain cases like fluoridation of drinking water or measles vaccination. Sometimes prevention can help buy healthy years of life, particularly during one's working years. However, if you think preventive care is going to produce the cash needed to fix some of the problems of our health care system, like covering the uninsured, it isn't. The true value of prevention is not in its cost savings ability, but in its potential to improve the quality and length of life—very important goals.

We end with an accolade to our friend Bill Crutchfield. He runs a small business with an incentive plan for every one of his employees to stay healthy. He does it, not because it will save a lot of money, but because it is the right thing to do.

7

MYTH: AMERICA WILL NOT RATION HEALTH CARE

The "R" word—"Rationing." No one wants to talk about it because it is the "third rail" of American health care politics: touch it and you are dead. Rationing is the opposite of the American dream; you know, that dream in which we can all have everything, like living forever (or, at least to well over 100) with good health and white teeth until the day we die. Mix that with a generation of us "Baby Boomers" who are used to having what we want when we want it. Therefore, rationing is not on anyone's radar screen, right? Wrong. Despite what we think, we cannot have it all, and we already do ration health care.

EARLY ATTEMPTS AT RATIONING IN THE UNITED STATES

A New Machine for Kidney Disease

Let's go back to the early 1960s when a new machine that provided "dialysis" for people with kidney failure was just becoming available. These machines took people who were otherwise certain to die, and kept them alive for long periods of time. But, the number of machines was severely limited and dialysis was extremely costly. Decisions had to be made as to who would be put on the machine, and live, and who would not be put on the machine, and die. Committees were formed of doctors, nurses, clergy, and others to help decide who should receive dialysis. They reviewed the "worthiness" of individuals to receive the service. While these committees tried, they became increasingly frustrated, and many simply threw up their hands and said they could not decide. So the federal government stepped in, and by the early 1970s, Congress approved dialysis for all those with kidney failure, and decided to pay for it through a relatively new health care program called "Medicare." Treatment for chronic kidney disease (for those of any age) was added to Medicare coverage largely because America was unable to ration health care. By the 1990s, the chronic kidney disease program used five percent of Medicare funds for less than one-half of one percent of Medicare's population, and today, this has risen to nine percent of Medicare payments. Please understand, this is not a negative commentary about the worthiness of treating kidney disease, but only a fact about our inability to make tough decisions regarding the availability of medical care, particularly when a new service is offered, the need is great, and patients demand it.

The Oregon Rationing Experiment

The next public attempt to ration health care was the state of Oregon's Medicaid program that went into effect in 1994. Oregon officials had determined that many of their citizens were going without needed medical care because they were uninsured and not eligible for Medicaid. They also knew that it would be impossible to provide every medical service for every uninsured person in the state, so Oregon policymakers proposed a plan that offered health coverage to those without insurance by enrolling them in a revised Medicaid program. The only way to pay for this new group of people was to limit, or ration, care. In 1989, the Oregon Health Services Commission was formed to create a list of approximately 700 medical conditions and their treatments. The list categorized the medical services as either "essential services" that prevented death with full recovery (for example, appendectomy), or as "very important services" where the treatment improved quality of life (for example, migraine), or as "services valuable to certain individuals" (for example, infertility services) or, lastly, whether the treatment had only "minimal effect" (for example, end-stage cancer).

Oregon Medicaid was then going to pay for treatment beginning at the top of the list covering essential services (such as the appendectomy) and continue funding medical care on down the list until the state Medicaid money ran out at the end of each year.

We have a lot to learn from what went on in this Oregon rationing experiment. First of all, no one could agree on how to do the ranking. They began using straightforward cost-effectiveness analysis (discussed in Chapter 3), but they could not agree on what should be considered "essential" and "very important." To "fix" the problem, they used focus groups made up from the general public to decide which services would be on the list. Interestingly, this selection process caused problems because two-thirds of the members of the focus groups were health care practitioners who often thought that the most important conditions to pay for were those most related to their area of practice, such as dentistry or certain types of medical care. For example, if a dentist led the group, preventive dental care was found toward the top of the list. In time, and to make up for a lack of a broad consensus, the commission produced the final list by doing what it thought was right. However, when the Oregon plan with its list of prioritized covered benefits was submitted to the federal government for approval in the summer of 1992, the plan was rejected on the grounds that it discriminated against people with disabilities (for example, highly expensive treatments for incurable cancer, the final stages of AIDS, or extremely premature infants with virtually no chance of survival), and violated the federal Americans with Disabilities Act. Nonetheless, two years later, under a different administration in Washington, the plan was approved.

The lesson of the Oregon "experiment" is that true rationing is easier in theory than in practice, given politics, patients, and physicians who want to make the system work only for them. Shortly after the program began, the system began to unravel. This failure resulted, in part, from the federal government requiring coverage of almost all services for certain groups (such as those with disabilities) as well as practitioners figuring how to get around the "rules," such as coding treatments for patients with multiple medical problems under categories that were covered even though they all might not have been covered individually. As a result, Oregon's rationing system did less rationing than expected, and in turn, provided less cost savings than projected. Net savings were only two percent after five years.

RATIONING AND INSURANCE COVERAGE

But, in truth, the United States *does* ration. Consider the following statement, found in many health insurance plans: "insurance companies do not pay for experimental treatment." On its surface, this exclusion seems reasonable. If a company wants to draw a line to limit services in an attempt to hold down costs, this is a place to start. But, we might ask, "experimental treatment" according to whom? In many cases, "experimental treatment" is decided by the medical director of an insurance company on the basis of, "I do not think there is enough evidence that it works." There is nothing necessarily wrong with that kind of determination as long as it is based on evidence, as long as it is not arbitrarily decided, and as long as other medical directors across the country use similar criteria to decide what is considered "experimental." Unfortunately, that is not always the case. Interpretations can vary about what therapies are medically necessary and when new treatments should be reclassified from "experimental" to "accepted medical practice." As a result, what services are actually covered varies greatly. For example, on the basis of the *same data* (in which a one percent improvement in mortality was found for a drug that cost $1,000 more than the current standard drug), an insurance company in one part of a large state decided to cover the drug, and the same company in another part of the state did not. This points up the variation in insurance coverage decisions, and, some would say, rationing by one and not the other.

Insurance companies ration coverage for mental health services because the chronic nature of the illnesses is extremely expensive. Additionally, the insurance companies can say that there is a difficulty in measuring clear outcomes of mental health services. Treatment of mental illness may not have an outcome that is "important" to insurance companies. Subjective measures such as "feeling better," or a better score on a depression scale before and after treatment may be difficult to translate into improved job performance. As discussed in Chapter 1, lost school days, juvenile incarceration, and absenteeism from work can each be based on social factors rather than, or in addition to, medical factors, and insurance companies can choose to deny coverage for mental health services on the basis that the problem lies outside the realm of "necessary medical care."

Some companies don't cover mental health at all, period. In a bit more subtle way, insurance companies ration by making employees pay higher "co-payments" (payment by the patient at the time of the service) for mental health services compared with other medical treatments covered under an insurance plan. Insurers also ration by covering only those services considered "biological," like schizophrenia or bipolar disorder.

In addition to rationing experimental treatments and mental health services, most insurance policies also have "preexisting condition" exclusions, which deny insurance coverage for medical conditions present at the time of employment. Generally, this denial of insurance coverage extends for a period of time, such as a year; during that year, there is no payment for treatments for the "pre-existing" condition like heart failure. But the company may also deny coverage without any time limit and can even completely exclude specific diseases, such as cancer (or as we have seen, mental illness), whether the person had the disease previously or not.

Other than simply saving on the cost of care for a year, insurance companies have another reason for pre-existing condition exclusions. Think about it: in the absence of pre-existing condition exclusions, patients could wait until they got sick before buying insurance. If this were allowed, few who were "well" would have insurance because they would simply wait until they needed it to buy it. Since the entire philosophy of insurance is pooling risk so the "well" subsidize the "sick," one important reason to have a preexisting condition exclusion is to cause "well" people to buy insurance before they are sick, to ensure coverage when they need it and to guarantee enough "well people" in the insurance pool. Of course, in situations where coverage is available for all (e.g., Medicare for those over sixty-five years of age), inducements such as preexisting condition exclusions are not necessary.

Finally, another rationing strategy used by insurance companies and employers is requiring patients to ration themselves. This type of self-rationing is just starting in a significant way with "high deductible" health plans. Consumers now decide how much health care they want and can afford. With a high deductible plan, the consumer pays for the first $1,000 to $2,000 (even $5,000) of yearly expenses (the deductible) before insurance kicks in. As we will see in Chapter 10, consumers may not always make the best decisions about their own rationing.

RATIONING AS A LACK OF ACCESS AND COVERAGE

The ultimate rationing tools in the U.S. are lack of health insurance coverage and lack of access to needed medical care. As we discussed in Chapter 1, "coverage" is defined as having health insurance, whether paid for by the employer, the government (Medicare, Medicaid, state or county hospital), or individually. We ration health care in this country by allowing forty-six million people to go without any insurance coverage.

As we will see in Chapter 14, the uninsured get about half the care of the insured, definitely a form of rationing. "Access" is defined as being able to see an appropriate practitioner at the appropriate time. Access is limited most obviously in the Medicaid program, where in some states as many as twenty-five percent of children who are eligible for Medicaid do not sign up. The reasons for this "lack of access" to health insurance through the Medicaid program may be because applicants (or their parents) are required to appear in person but have no transportation; or they do not have the appropriate documentation to prove how poor they are, or they may be unable to complete an application form that may extend up to sixteen pages. This is also discussed further in Chapter 14.

THE REST OF THE WORLD ALSO RATIONS

We are not alone; every country in the world rations, but each in a different way. Many countries have a limited list of drugs that government insurance will pay for; if the drug is not on that list, there is no payment. Some countries limit these drugs "because their effectiveness has not yet been proven," in other words, they are still experimental (we have heard those words before). In England and Australia, mathematical cost-effectiveness analysis is actually used, just like the design of the Oregon rationing experiment, and some drugs are not available because their effectiveness does not justify the cost. The most open form of rationing has been used in certain European countries where, for example, dialysis was not available to anyone over the age of sixty-five. This rationing practice has been replaced by more quiet agreements between families and physicians that consider the patient's quality of life. As we will see in Chapter 19, such discussions seem to be less common in the United

States because of our values that seem to require a great deal of medical care, even at the end of life.

The most common form of rationing throughout the developed world is limited access to health services through a "waiting list." Each country's health care system has an overall budget. This limited funding pays, for example, a certain amount to each hospital each year. The hospital has enough supplies for a certain number of operations. It becomes the problem of the hospital and physicians to decide the types and number of procedures that can be done each year within the budget. Since there are generally more procedures required than money available, less seriously ill patients are "delayed until next year" and are put on waiting lists. Clearly, some life saving procedures such as cancer surgery and coronary artery bypass surgery cannot wait (and may be done relatively quickly or receive high priority on the waiting list), whereas other, more elective procedures, such as hip replacement, are moved further down the list. While it is true that some patients die "while waiting on the waiting list," it is more common for patients to have a lower quality of life while they are waiting for their procedures.

Every other country provides access for the wealthy by having a second "private" system. In the majority of countries, one can wait for months to see a physician in the public system, but can have an appointment, perhaps even the next day, in the private system. Patients in other countries are now buying health insurance so that if they get sick, they can be seen in the private system. Even Canada, which has historically not allowed private insurance, is going this way: just this past year, a Montreal businessman sued and won the right to purchase private health insurance for a hip replacement so that he wouldn't have to wait a year for the surgery. This ruling is expected to allow broader private health services in the country. Sound familiar? In the United States, we began with private health insurance and then built Medicare and Medicaid to cover those who fell outside the employer-sponsored health insurance model. In most other countries, they began with public health insurance and are now progressing to private health insurance.

Clearly, in the United States, virtually any form of rationing for the eighty-four percent who have health insurance has so far been unacceptable to us. Rationing would mean that some services would not be available; this means that not only does the patient not get something, but also the provider or the supplier loses income since that service is no longer available. We want everything. We want it now, and we will initiate a lawsuit if we think it is available and we do not get it.

WHAT CAN WE DO?

How will we deal with the ever-increasing availability of new diagnostic tests and treatments that are increasingly expensive? In the short term, we will make every attempt to avoid rationing, and, for a while, we will continue to pay more. We will continue to foot the bill rather than take less or wait longer.

We believe that eventually there will be guidelines to decide what should be covered. Ideally, the services that are covered should provide a reasonable baseline for every American, one that we would be proud to tell our friends around the world, but one that is not excessive. We should make the services cover those treatments for which there is evidence that the service is beneficial (so called "evidence-based benefits"). In some cases, because there will not be studies available, expert opinion (such as that currently found in many national practice guidelines) will have to suffice.

However, even the list of truly beneficial services is likely to be unaffordable at some point, and then the really hard work will begin. A system such as the one tried in Oregon will likely be developed using a combination of mathematical cost effectiveness and common sense, generating a list of covered services. Payment for treatments related to diseases linked to self-defeating behavior such as smoking and overeating, as well as "futile" care at the extremes of life (as discussed in Chapter 4), will have to be balanced against paying for other effective treatments. Who will make the decisions about which medical services are "essential"? Because it is important to take such decisions out of the realm of politics, a completely independent group like the Federal Reserve may need to be established. Broad decisions regarding the insurance coverage of essential medical services cannot be reached by individuals, either by the physicians treating patients or by the patients themselves, since, at the individual level, everyone will always want everything. However, this doesn't mean that physician and patient input is not important: in determining what is "essential" we will need to gather information from many types of health practitioners as well as patients, the general public, ethicists, and social scientists to help develop the methodology and conduct the research to assess the medical evidence. Whether it is more important to maximize the benefit to a single identified patient who is ill (e.g., "my son") or whether it is more important to maximize the good of a larger number of people (e.g., "the community"), with the same number of life years saved, are examples of the kind of questions and trade-offs that will have to be discussed.

Once the list of services is developed, the budget will determine what is covered, whether it is business saying this is all they will pay, or through government programs such as Medicare. How much medical care we can ultimately afford to pay for is likely to be defined by how much waste we can eliminate in the current system and how much we, as a country, decide to continue to spend on medical care. If the services that are considered "essential" cannot be covered, then there are really only two choices: increase the amount people are willing to pay, or further ration the care.

Because this is America, those who can pay will be able to buy more care than those who cannot pay. This disparity is not unethical as long as we define an "adequate" baseline of care and provide it to everyone. Unfortunately, the definition of "adequate" depends upon where you stand. No matter what, we will eventually need to come to grips with the fact that we cannot all have it all.

III

QUALITY: THE MYTHS OF GOOD CARE

MYTH: SCIENCE DRIVES MOST MEDICAL DECISIONS

HOW ARE MEDICAL DECISIONS MADE?

Less than fifteen percent of medical decisions are based on "appropriate evidence." Now that we have your attention, let us explain why this is so. Up until about forty years ago, medical decisions were based on clinical experience, information in textbooks, or by asking colleagues and experts. For years, quality was indeed in the eye of the practicing physician and quality of care was taken for granted.

This model began to unravel in the early 1970s when a growing body of research showed that doctors across the country were treating patients with the same diseases in different ways and that no one really knew what was the "best" treatment. The "shot heard round the world" came in 1989 when the results of a large clinical trial called the Cardiac Arrhythmia Suppression Trial (CAST) were published. This study was designed to give information about and help some of the 400,000 people in the United States who die suddenly each year because of coronary heart disease. Before the CAST trial, doctors knew that after a heart attack, people often died suddenly. They also knew that the greater the number of extra "premature" heartbeats that patients with heart disease had, the more likely they were to die suddenly. In an effort to address this problem, the CAST trial was designed to see which of the medicines used would decrease the extra beats most effectively and prevent sudden death. Twenty-seven clinical centers around the country enrolled 4,400 patients who had previously had heart attacks and gave them either a placebo (sugar pill) or one of the three drugs used to treat premature heartbeats. The clinical trial was stopped early because it was clear that one group was doing much better than the others. When they looked at the groups, the one doing the best was the group receiving the "placebo"—all the actual drugs were making the patients worse! This trial showed us that conventional wisdom in medicine is not always right and that currently held medical assumptions need testing.

As a result, the "double blind, placebo controlled, randomized clinical trial" then became the gold standard for determining the effective use of diagnostic and therapeutic technologies and for improving medical practice. Those words mean:

1. Double blind: neither the doctor nor the patient knows whether they are getting the treatment (e.g., the pill that is being tested). While it does not occur commonly, it is possible for doctors to be biased in how they report data if they know which patient is receiving an experimental drug for a particular treatment. Similarly, patients, if they know they are receiving the drug, could be "optimistic" in reporting their symptoms because they want a drug to work. Therefore, trials should be "blinded to both doctors and patients."
2. Trials should also be "placebo controlled," which means that one group of patients receives a "placebo" or sugar pill while the other group receives the experimental drug to be sure that the observed effects are actually due to the drug and not simply the result of taking a pill.
3. "Randomized" means that patients are assigned completely at random as to whether they get the experimental drug or not. Patients who are participating in these trials are counseled completely before participating and sign detailed forms giving their consent, recognizing that they have a 50-50 chance of receiving either the placebo or the treatment drug.

We have also learned that drug trials need to be carried out for long periods of time (in the best case over several years) to demonstrate how well drugs work in practice. An example of this came a few years ago when we discovered that some of the newer (and more expensive) drugs for blood pressure control are actually no better than the older, less expensive ones that have been traditionally used.

PRACTICE GUIDELINES AND EVIDENCE-BASED MEDICINE

The CAST trial and other studies demonstrated that there is a need for good evidence to inform medical decision making and improve quality care, but there are other reasons as well: doing the "wrong thing" is wasteful, and costs more. Only a small percentage of our medical decisions are based on these kinds of large-scale clinical trials, mainly because they are not always practical and because they can be extremely expensive. For example, in children, only eleven percent of guidelines for recommended treatment are based on randomized clinical trials, while almost three-quarters come from the less dependable "expert opinion," where there may be varying judgments. Many medical decisions are based on other types of scientific research findings that permit important conclusions—but can be more questioned by physicians than the randomized controlled trial. We also know that some decisions will always be based on how physicians have traditionally been taught that something "seems to work" based on the experience of their teachers. Medical training has historically relied on mentors' experiences, but unfortunately, different people with different experiences may teach physicians—thus teaching to practice differently on similar patients. The cycle continues when young physicians develop their own "experience," which is certainly neither randomized nor controlled.

For all of these reasons, there is tremendous variation in how patients are treated. In Chapter 3, we introduced you to the data that demonstrated extreme variation throughout the country. For example, patients with lung disease who live in Boston are hospitalized 2.2 times as often as for similar patients who live in New Haven, Connecticut. In fact, for patients with hip fractures and heart attacks, "doing less" is associated with better survival. How can this be? When a greater number of physicians are involved in a given patient's care, greater numbers of tests are performed, and hospital stays are longer. Patients who have longer hospitalizations have higher rates of infection. Having a large number of physicians involved in the care of the same patient is likely to cause communication problems, certainly making the process inefficient, but also, in some cases, making the care less effective: as the number of physicians involved increases, each thinks the other one is doing something. Additionally, when too many tests are used, they may turn up "problems" that require further tests to prove that the problems are not important.

So, what are we to do? Physicians need to develop data on how to practice efficiently, and agree on best practice. Recognizing this problem, physicians have been developing "practice guidelines." These are "rules of thumb" for how to handle the most common illnesses. They are prepared primarily by national societies of physicians (such as the American College of Cardiology) who have groups of experts convene to produce guidelines indicating, for example, who *definitely* does or does not need a pacemaker (when the data are sufficient to demonstrate that), or who *probably* does or does not need a pacemaker based on their collective judgment (when the data are less than complete). These guidelines are revised frequently and constitute the best available information for physicians. Patients treated according to the guidelines have better outcomes. In fact, as we will see in Chapter 9, many "quality measures" of physician and hospital performance are based on how well the practice guidelines are followed.

Translating Evidence into Medical Practice

Why wouldn't physicians follow guidelines? Most often it is because the physician has not been able to "keep up" with new information about treating a medical condition. An important advance provided by computerized electronic medical records is the inclusion of practice guidelines. For example, the physician types as a diagnosis "slow heart rate," and the national guidelines for "who needs a pacemaker" are displayed on the screen—since that is a treatment for "slow heart rate." The other reason that guidelines may not be followed is that the physician does not agree with the guidelines—he or she "knows better" (remember, their "professor" may have taught them differently!). That may be the case, but it also may not be a valid argument. The most important and valid reason for not following the guidelines is that they do not apply to that particular patient. In many cases, this decision could be correct. Practice guidelines are created for the "most typical" patient and, in some cases, the physician may feel that the guideline is not a good "fit." The patient may be too old, too sick, have complicating factors, or have personal preferences that make implementation of the guideline less appropriate. The probability that physicians will follow practice guidelines is about fifty percent, a number disappointing to those who believe that practice guidelines will reduce variation and tie medical decision-making to evidence. Ultimately, the guidelines need to get better and better so that they apply to increasing numbers of patients.

Unfortunately, even the most well-used and accepted guidelines cannot teach us when to ignore the guidelines. This is where the "art" of medicine becomes so important: we must know when to apply and when not to apply the guidelines. Innovation is then required on the part of a physician to know what to do when the guidelines do not apply. As we will see in Chapter 9, most physicians do well with routine cases, but one measure of an outstanding physician is how well they do with the cases that are *not* routine. Unifying the "art" of clinical judgment with the science of well-reasoned guidelines is optimal, and increasingly, decision-making will be based on evidence as well as experience. It is likely that with computerized electronic medical records, vastly improved data will be developed to show what works for patients. As these patient data (as well as "exceptions" where guidelines may not apply as reported by physicians) are continually used to update the guidelines, they will become more specific to individual patients so that more "acceptable evidence" will be available for physicians to use in treating their patients. As more and more physicians find that guidelines are relevant for their individual patients, variation in treatment patterns and outcomes will decrease and results will improve. By blending an experienced clinician's intuition with evidence, we will be able to increase the fifteen percent portion of medicine that is based on "acceptable evidence." But even as the science improves, the need for the "art" of medicine will remain.

9

MYTH: HIGH QUALITY CARE CANNOT BE DEFINED

TOWARD A DEFINITION OF QUALITY

Sit around a dinner table and ask, "What makes a good doctor?" You might think that this would ruin the party, but it doesn't. Try it.

The first half of the people around the table are generally consistent: "the doctor talks to me"; "knows my family"; "easy to make an appointment with." By the time five people have answered in a similar way, it is then worthwhile to ask, gently, "Doesn't it matter if the doctor makes you better?" Answer: "Oh, we *assumed* that!" Wrong.

Quality does differ among practitioners, and quality does matter, in areas very important to all of us like the treatment of cancer, kidney disease, high blood pressure, and what happens when we have a heart attack. According to the Institute of Medicine, quality health care contains six important aims, or elements:

1. *Patient-centeredness.* Does the physician relate well to the patient, consider the patient's wishes and values, and keep the patient informed? This is the part of quality that our dinner guests referred to above. One measure of this is patient satisfaction, often measured through patient surveys.

2. *Timeliness.* Can the patient be seen in a "timely" way? Or, in other words, when the referring physician and the patient want to be seen?

But in addition to respecting the patient's satisfaction and schedule, there are other dimensions that indicate quality:

3. *Effectiveness.* Is the correct treatment done and is it done correctly? Is the treatment given appropriately to those who need it and not given to those who don't? What are the results of treatment—i.e., did the patient get better?

4. *Efficiency.* Are resources such as equipment, supplies, and people's time being wasted? Waste is, by definition, bad quality, since un-needed tests and treatments are expensive, inconvenient, and possibly even dangerous. One study suggests that twenty-two percent of sick adults in America had been sent for the same tests within a few days of each other by different health care professionals. This type of waste is "inefficient" since the money can be used in better ways.

5. *Equity.* Does everyone have a fair opportunity to have health care of the same high quality regardless of gender, ethnicity, geographic loca-tion, socioeconomic status, and whether one has health insurance? In other words, are we treating patients with the same diseases the same way, for example, no matter what their race? Currently, we do not. Health disparities exist in the United States. For example, Caucasian life expectancy for both sexes is 77.7 years, yet for African Americans it is only 72.3 years. For virtually all forms of cancer, those with lower income have higher mortality that those with higher income. Same for where you live: death rates for children and young adults ages one to twenty-four are highest in rural counties, and, as we discussed in Chapter 1, the life expectancy in Harlem in New York City is lower than the life expectancy in Bangladesh. And the data are similar for the uninsured, a topic we'll discuss in chapters 14 through 18.

6. *Safety.* Health professionals make mistakes? It has been estimated that 98,000 patients die in hospitals *each year* because of medical er-rors, about 300 people per day. That is not an easy number to relate to but it is the equivalent of a jumbo jet crash *per day*, and three times the number of people who die on highways each year. Every day two patients have either the wrong limb amputated or the wrong kidney

taken out. Approximately one to three percent of all hospital admissions will result in death or harm from injuries, not from their disease, but from the medical care itself. Preventable infections acquired in hospitals are estimated to cost $4.5 billion per year, and contribute to more than 88,000 deaths—one death every six minutes in the United States. Why? One problem is we health care professionals don't check ourselves and don't ask for help often enough. We have much to learn from the airline industry that has popularized pre-flight safety checklists, where team behavior is the norm, and the co-pilot is expected to question the pilot. These observations and practices have led to changed behavior in the operating room where now the surgeon (no less strong willed than pilots) must check with the anesthesiologist and the nurse to be sure, for example, that the correct side of the body is being operated on (such as in the removal of the correct kidney). We know that many errors are related to poor communication between health care providers and their patients. The patient and family must become more a part of the overall care team: all of us should question each other to improve care and help change the processes that currently allow too many avoidable medical injuries.

Thus, we have defined quality and its six elements. As patients work their way through the maze of quality and what it means to them, each patient as an individual will need to rank each of the six elements in order of importance when choosing a physician or a hospital in which to have a procedure; ideally every one is important, but, for example, some may sacrifice timeliness and feel that waiting an extra month is worth seeing a super-specialist.

THE PATIENT'S GUIDE TO QUALITY

Right now, it takes work to find data about quality. If you want quality information about individual physicians, the data are scarce, but are becoming more available every day. Most health plans provide patient satisfaction data at least for all the doctors as a group, and, increasingly, by individual physicians. If a patient is relatively healthy, it is likely that how the doctor relates to them (patient-centeredness and timeliness) are going to be high on the list of importance, and these are well measured by patient satisfaction data.

The Internet provides a convenient gateway for patients and providers alike when looking for quality measures. For example, Healthgrades.com provides "quality reports" on 600,000 physicians, with information on medical training, board certification, and any disciplinary action taken in the past five years by state or federal authorities. The "effectiveness" quality element discussed above is likely related to board certification. In today's world, board certification, for example, internal medicine, and sub-board certification, for instance, cardiology, is an indication that a physician had to pass a broad examination assessing what they know. Many boards and sub-boards require continuing education and examination in order to maintain certification. Therefore, up-to-date board certification is a general indication that a physician has kept up with current practice standards.

Education and Training. While individuals who train in "big name" programs may be excellent, so are those who trained in less well-known programs, and so information about education alone may not be very helpful when making a decision about who may or may not be the best doctor.

Government Disciplinary Actions. Most definitely, if an individual has lost his or her license to practice, this is a huge red flag (potentially in "effectiveness" or "safety"), and a patient would want to know that. However, given today's high rates of malpractice suits, it is not *necessarily* an indicator of a low quality physician if he or she has been sued a number of times or even has had judgments against them—but it is worth asking the physician whether the law suit was in the area relating to your disease.

Grades, Rankings, and Report Cards

Data on outcomes (e.g., death, or complications of an operation) from the care delivered by individual physicians is becoming more commonly available. The best publicized individual physician outcome data are in the New York State Cardiovascular Surgery database through the New York State Department of Health (www.health.state.ny.us/nysdeoh/comsumer.heart). Every surgeon in the state that does coronary bypass surgery is included. But, this database illustrates the two major problems with individual physician outcome data:

1. For physicians with a small number of patients, the data may not tell the story. This is just the law of small numbers that if you have data

based on three cases, it will be less reliable than data obtained from 100 cases. However, the mere fact that a surgeon does less than the average number of cases *may* be a sign that he or she is not experienced, or does not get referrals (for any number of reasons, such as poor results in other procedures that are *not* listed, or even the physician's personality); low numbers of procedures may have nothing to do with quality and perhaps only be an indication of someone who recently moved to the area and is beginning to accumulate data. In general, physicians who perform procedures (for example, surgeons and interventional cardiologists) have better results the more they do.

2. Data on outcomes (such as death after heart surgery) must be compared only among patients with a similar severity of the medical problem. For example, all coronary artery bypass operations are not the same: if one patient has one diseased vessel and another has five diseased vessels, the second patient has a more severe problem, carries a higher risk of death from the operation, and the long-term results may be different. Higher risk also occurs if the patient has had coronary bypass surgery previously or if the patient is very old. It is important to find out if the data on the individual surgeon are compared for similar severity. If the data are not, the surgeons who operated on tougher cases and sicker patients will have significantly higher mortality rates. This does not make them "lower quality" physicians; it just may mean they are operating on sicker people. Therefore, whether a patient is reading the "report card" in the newspaper or asking a surgeon, what is important to know is at a minimum how many of these procedures the surgeon has done compared with the average and compared with the five physicians who have done it most frequently (for example, if the average surgeon has done twenty cases, and the surgeon you are considering has done thirty, that may seem good until you find out that the five who do it most frequently have each done two hundred).

One other problem with this type of data is that they are presented statistically: percent mortality (death) or percent complications (what went badly). Unless the patient is a statistician, trying to figure out whether one surgeon's statistics are better than another is difficult at best. The best way to approach this is to: look for the results for your exact problem for the average surgeon and for the five best surgeons in the country. If the patient has a choice, it is best to be with those closer to the top but at least halfway between the average and the top. It is also worthwhile to know how unusual or complex the patient's case is. Again, it is always best to go for the best, but the more unusual or difficult your case, the more important it would be to choose a physician closer to the top in terms of numbers and results, and are more likely to be able to deal with unusual and complicated cases.

So, it is important to look at these types of "report card" data when choosing a physician for a specific procedure, but remember, the information is often limited.

Data for hospitals are much more available. We have reviewed two websites that are likely to continue to provide data long into the future. The first is the Joint Commission on Accreditation of Healthcare Organizations (www.jcaho.org), the oldest and largest non-governmental agency that accredits hospitals and ranks their safety and quality. The second is the site for the federal government's Centers for Medicare and Medicaid Services, (www.hospitalcompare.cms.gov). At present, both of these groups rank heart attack care and heart failure care in a large number of hospitals, and JCAHO also ranks the quality of care during pregnancy. Both websites give a summary compared to average performance (e.g., "better than average, average, or worse than average"). For the data they consider to be most important, they use performance measures of the type that we discussed in Chapter 8 that relate to the percent of patients for whom care guidelines are followed. For example, what percent of patients who have heart attacks followed the guideline that said to prescribe aspirin at the time of discharge from the hospital after their heart attack (aspirin helps prevent heart attacks by slightly thinning blood). They display what percentage of patients get aspirin in the average hospital and what percent get aspirin in the top ten percent of hospitals. Clearly, most patients will not be interested in the specific measures, but simply looking in general at the fact that most measures for the specific illness are "better than average" should be important. Hospitals that are outstanding in one disease may not be in all diseases, and it is important to look for the specific condition. If data are not available, consider an overall rating of hospitals such as can be found at www.100tophospitals.com.

Increasingly, individuals are being called upon to choose a "health plan," usually an insurance company with specific types of coverage. Most commonly, an employer provides a set of health plan choices to employees, and each plan will have access to particular "providers," a term that includes physicians and other practitioners as well as hospitals. The National Committee for Quality Assurance—NCQA—is a private, not-for-profit organization whose mission is to improve the quality of health care by providing understandable information to help inform consumer and employer choice. The NCQA accredits and rates health plans (mostly Health Maintenance Organizations) against more than sixty different standards that measure performance in five broad categories:

1. *Access and Services*: Do health plan members have access to the care and service they need? Does the health plan resolve grievances fairly and quickly? This measure includes plan administrative services such as how long a patient has to wait for an appointment or the number of rings until the telephone is answered.
2. *Qualified Providers*: Does the health plan thoroughly check the credentials of all its providers? This measure would include board certification, disciplinary actions, and patient satisfaction ratings.
3. *Staying Healthy*: Does the health plan provide appropriate screening tests and immunizations for the members?
4. *Getting Better*: How well does the plan care for people when they become sick, such as providing appropriate treatment for children with upper respiratory infections?
5. *Living with Illness*: How well does the plan help people manage chronic illness, for example, blood pressure control in those patients who are hypertensive or comprehensive care for diabetic patients?

The concepts that apply to doctors and hospitals also apply to health plans: in general, the health plans with the higher number of people enrolled generally have better results. In fact, since most of the measures reported on public report cards for health plans and hospitals involve physicians, the "hospital and health plan measures" reasonably reflect the performance of the physicians working there. We have seen that quality data are increasingly available and increasingly understandable. But how much do patients really look at the data? Do we care? Are we good market-directed consumers? Read on in Chapter 10.

10

MYTH: CONSUMERS CAN MAKE THE BEST DECISIONS ABOUT THEIR MEDICAL CARE

HOW DO CONSUMERS MAKE DECISIONS?

We consumers buy all kinds of things. We read *Consumer Reports*, read the instructions about how to use things, and we make choices. In medical care, we are not as likely to do as well in our decisions as we do with shirts, cars, and auto insurance. The shirt is absolutely clear; we can try it on, see how it looks, know exactly what it costs, and even bring it back tomorrow if we don't like it. The car is sort of like the shirt; some can even be returned within thirty days, but we don't know how well it was constructed or how long it will last. Yes, there is a warranty, but it seems like the one thing that goes wrong with the car is not covered by the warranty, and we sure didn't know *that* in advance. When we are getting the oil changed in our automobile, we look for the advertisement with the lowest price; when deciding where to take the car for repairs, we either go back to the dealer, take it to a nationally recognized chain, or go where our brother-in-law takes his car. If needed, we ask them to "fix the knock in my engine" and rarely hang around for an explanation of what is wrong. If we find out that the other place charged our friend less for the same problem and the car seems fixed, we go to the other place the next time. Similarly, when it comes to car insurance, we wonder how much coverage we should have. What can we afford? Should we be careful of the fine print on page fifty-six of the policy? Forget it, we think, "The companies may have flashy logos, but they really aren't that different,"—or are they? They all pay quickly and completely, don't they? What can we do if they don't pay?

Sound familiar? The point is we make decisions every day without complete information and on "faith" that the result will turn out well. We do the same with medical care, although it often seems like we have even less information than we do for our other day-to-day decisions. In fact, we may not. Do the repair shops post their results for "fixing unknown engine knocks"? Do the car insurers tell you "the percent of claims paid in three days"?

MAKING DECISIONS ABOUT MEDICAL CARE

So how are consumers going to make decisions about their medical care, and how successful will they be? In the end, they may find that the way they make health decisions may be a lot closer to the way they choose shirts, cars, and auto insurance. For example:

1. *Personal Health Care*. We ignore all kinds of information about smoking and obesity leading to diabetes, despite the fact that we know better. That behavior is *not* due to a lack of understandable information; more likely it reflects how tough it is to change bad habits. Chapter 6 presented information about how people with chronic illness often stop taking their medication, and fail to show up for appointments. At least half of patients fail to follow their doctor's recommended treatment. When you think of it that way, consumers are not directing their own health care so well, are they? How can physicians help patients make good decisions about their health?

   (a) First of all, physicians should work with patients to create "patient practice guidelines" to indicate when, generally speaking, a physician visit is needed and why—and even when a visit may not be necessary. Doing less based on good evidence does not mean withholding appropriate care, but rather practicing good medicine. And, patient-centered care, which we discussed in the last chapter, requires a trusted partnership between the physician and patient. Physicians can also work to tighten physician practice guidelines to reduce waste, as discussed in Chapter 3.

(b) Second, money seems to drive some people, so an increased cigarette tax, a proposed tax on fatty foods or sugary drinks, or increasing insurance premiums on those with clearly self-defeating lifestyles may be required. We know that with increased taxes on both cigarettes and alcohol, we have seen reduced consumption over the last decade; nineteen states currently have taxes on particular junk foods such as soda. Most U.S. residents believe smokers and heavy drinkers should pay a different level for their health insurance. And, while some Americans are concerned about negative measures to reduce unhealthy behaviors, most agree that at the very least, positive incentives from employers or insurers, such as free fitness programs, should be given to induce healthier lifestyles.

2. *Medical decisions.* Patients must always be informed. They should "direct" their own care when there are a number of ways to decide or when personal preferences will make a difference. For example, the decision whether to have a wound sutured is not an option, although the risk of infection should be explained. On the other hand, in many cases of prostate cancer and breast cancer, the likelihood of long-term survival is similar with different medical treatments; however, the after-effects of the different procedures (for example, impotence after prostate surgery) are likely to be viewed entirely differently by different individuals and, in that case, individual preferences should be the deciding factor in the decision.

3. *Decisions on Physician, Hospital, or Health Plan.* The patient must be comfortable with his or her physician. Much of a patient's comfort with a physician is personal interaction, but the patients should also have available to them certain facts about the physician, such as board certification, and, as discussed in Chapter 9, the physician's history of success with certain procedures, including rates of death and complications when compared with other physicians who perform the same procedure. If a patient requires hospitalization, it is worthwhile to see if there are hospital ratings of "less than expected" (meaning that they are in the bottom half), and if so, pay particular attention to those as they relate to the patient's specific illness.

4. *Benefits*. Generally, this involves determining how much health care the patient wants. The choice can be broken down into five questions:

   (a) *How much "choice" is important to me?* Choosing one's own physician seems to be important to many people. Interestingly, the way doctors are chosen most commonly is to ask one's neighbors or colleagues at work shortly after a move to a new town. Then when a doctor is found, the patient asks the doctor about other doctors for referral. What seems to matter most is keeping the physicians that the patient likes. Whether the patient has access to a particular physician is likely to be an important factor in choosing the health benefit plan. Having access to an outstanding hospital or medical center may be additionally important to some who already have a history of illness.

   (b) *How likely is the patient to need medical care in the next year?* If one is twenty-six years old and a single man the answer is "not very likely"—not the case for a twenty-six-year-old woman who could become pregnant. And don't forget automobile and skiing accidents: insurance coverage is still essential no matter how old one is. However, if one is fifty-six, has had a heart attack, and is taking medication, the answer is "more likely."

   (c) *What services should be covered?* This is likely related as well to how sick the patient is, but consumers also are concerned about cost. Is it important to that patient to have mental health and eye care as covered services? If so, the insurance plan may be more expensive.

   (d) *How much risk is the person willing to take?* If one is a "risk taker" and fairly healthy, then choosing a "bare minimum" plan may be fine, although bare minimum plans rarely cover preventive care, and going without preventive care can cause problems later.

   (e) *How much money does the person want to spend?* Clearly, the more the person is willing to spend, the greater choice of benefits, physicians, and hospitals. The amount of the premium is usually related to the amount of the "deductible," which is the amount paid out of pocket before insurance starts to pay. As a general rule, the higher the deductible (e.g., going from $500 to $2,000), the lower the total premium.

CONSUMER-DIRECTED HEALTH CARE AND HIGH DEDUCTIBLE PLANS

In the case of "high deductible" health plans, the individual pays the first big chunk of medical expenses (often around $2,000) out of his or her pocket up front. This trend, often called "consumer directed healthcare" requires consumers (who later become patients) to make decisions about how best to spend that first $2,000. Sometimes they don't have a choice as to what to spend it on, such as if a serious medical event happens, but often they do. Should they spend it on dental care or a mammogram? What about that annual physical? How will they decide? Most studies have shown that when patients have to pay for their own care, they do with less, which may be helpful in eliminating waste, but also limits necessary care. In these kinds of cases, physicians can help with guidelines for patients, but there always remains the concern that patients, when choosing among other competing basic needs (such as rent, food, and bills), will forgo appropriate physician visits and tests, as well as important preventive care, when money is involved—the data say so. This is particularly bad for those who are low income or chronically ill, but it is true for others as well: under High Deductible Health Plans, the long-term health of Americans could suffer if individuals do not spend their own money (before they reach their deductibles) appropriately on prevention and other necessary health care. But it may take a long time for the effects of the lack of appropriate care to become apparent; for example, if women do not get Pap smears or mammograms, the cancer may not appear for five to ten years—and that's when we may all wake up and see that these plans have actually caused harm.

Patients must get information. But it is clear that some want a lot of information and some want a little; for some patients, understanding why a blood test of liver function is needed for someone taking a statin may be similar to an individual understanding why the oil in their car needs to be changed at 30,000 miles. As of today, most want their information from their doctor: in a recent survey asking patients where they would look for information and what information sources they trusted, a clear majority (seventy percent) responded they would ask a health care professional for specific information about a medical problem, and almost nine out of ten (eighty-eight percent) responded that their most trusted information source was their health care professional. The majority doesn't want the Internet.

While many may say this will change over time, it may not. A large number of patients prefer to seek advice and assistance from their doctor. To get back to our car analogy, consider this: the website http://www.Carcare.org advocates a "consumer-directed" approach to caring for your car. The website advises that "taking an active role in maintaining your vehicle is the best way to avoid costly repairs down the road." Sound familiar to the advice to get a flu shot, a mammogram, or visit the dentist? *Carcare.org* goes on to say that "many drivers tend to stall when it comes to keeping up with some everyday auto-basics," and cites the number of vehicles with low or dirty engine oil (thirty-eight percent), low tire pressure (fifty-four percent), or dirty air filters (sixteen percent). And yet, even with the evidence, how many consumers actually heed that advice about "preventive maintenance" about either their cars or their bodies? So, in addition to caring for the "informed" consumer, we must also be prepared for the response of the consumer-patient who has little interest or motivation to direct their health care and says to the doctor (as they would say to the mechanic for the oil change or transmission trouble), "fix it, don't tell me how, just fix it."

MYTH: FEWER DOCTORS WILL BE NEEDED AS MEDICINE CHANGES

CAN YOU SEE YOUR DOCTOR?

Can you get an appointment with your doctor tomorrow morning? How about in a month? Do you think this is because doctors *like* to make you wait? They are booked up because there are too few physicians, particularly in some areas of the country and in some medical specialties. And it is going to get worse.

There has been a recent reluctance to deal with physician workforce issues because every time in the past twenty years that a surplus or shortage of doctors has been predicted, the opposite has occurred. Take for example the last predictions made during the early 1990s during the growth of the Healthcare Maintenance Organizations (HMO). Because of the supposed "efficiencies" that HMOs created by using a "gatekeeper" model (in which primary care physicians were the "gatekeepers" requiring permission for the patient to see a specialist), it was argued that HMOs could be used as models to predict the appropriate number of physicians required. As a result, the number of physicians estimated to be needed for the future predicted a surplus. At the same time, because of the belief in the gatekeeper model, experts were predicting a shortage of "generalist" physicians like family practitioners, general internists, obstetrician-gynecologists, and general pediatricians. Recommendations advised that fifty percent of new physicians should enter these generalist disciplines and fifty percent should enter specialties (such as cardiology).

Well, the gatekeeper model disappeared as Americans insisted on having more freedom of choice about selecting their physicians and about having more direct access to specialists. The ratio of 50-50 (which made about as much sense as the ratio of U.S. Senators to Congressmen) was never achieved. The "generalist" area of family medicine is the only true "generalist": general internal medicine deals only with adults, pediatrics deals only with children, and obstetrics/gynecology, only women. So lumping those four medical disciplines never made sense, just as lumping all specialists doesn't make sense either: the need for plastic surgeons may not be the same as the need for cardiologists. A better way to plan for an adequate physician workforce is to design a formula that relates the numbers and types of physicians within a given geographic area and population. In this way, we would know what kinds of physicians are needed where. This is important because many Americans live in geographic regions where they lack access to physicians. A ratio of less than one physician to 3,500 persons is designated as a "health professional shortage area." These areas may be urban or rural areas. At present, over twenty percent of the U.S. population lives in an area designated as a health professional shortage area. These areas have traditionally and continue to need all types of health care practitioners, but, now, increasingly, they need specialist physicians.

What data do we have about the need for generalist and specialist physicians? Twelve states report some physician shortages now or expect shortages within the next few years. How long it takes to get an appointment to see a physician is not a bad way to get at a region's supply and demand. In a 2004 survey looking at wait times in fifteen big U.S. cities, average wait times for appointments to see skin cancer, heart, and knee specialists were three to four weeks, even when medical problems were suspected or injuries had occurred. On the "supply" side, seventy-one percent of recruiters for physicians say that for cardiologists, demand "far exceeds supply"; seventy-four percent of individuals finishing their cardiology training have five or more job offers. Cardiology is clearly telling us we have a problem with a physician shortage now, and so far ten other generalist and specialist physician groups are experiencing the same trends (e.g., general internal medicine, dermatology, allergy, radiology), which leads to the conclusion that over the next several years, the shortage of physicians will worsen; the current twelve states (e.g., Massachusetts, Texas, California, Mississippi) declaring physician shortages are likely to be joined by most of the others.

When we compare the United States with other countries in physician-to-population ratios, the U.S. is ranked thirteenth from the top out of twenty countries in the Organization for Economic Cooperation and Development (OECD). The physician-to-population ratio stands at 264 physicians per 100,000 population in the U.S., while the average for the OECD is 326.

TRENDS IN PHYSICIAN SUPPLY AND DEMAND: SUPPLY

Medical schools in the United States graduate a total of about 16,000 students a year, a number that has remained stable for more than two decades. There are approximately 23,000 post–medical school residency positions that last for three to eight years. We make up the difference between the number of U.S. medical graduates and residents by bringing into the U.S. approximately 7,000 physicians who graduate from overseas medical schools. Less than twenty percent of the international medical graduates return home, so each year, approximately 22,000 physicians finish their medical training residencies and enter practice in the United States. Over the past five years, the overall physician supply in the U.S. has grown only slightly (by eight percent), but when seen in relation to the U.S. population growth, the ratio of physicians to patients has grown half that much—four percent.

What do we know of the future? For the last several years, approximately fifty percent of physicians entering practice are women. Female physicians at present work about twenty percent fewer hours than men, and they will represent forty-five percent of practicing physicians by 2020; this is not to say that women should work longer hours, but that different work patterns require different workforce planning. In a recent study, sixty-four percent of *both* men and women say they will reduce hours they work over the next decade. This is not surprising. In addition to lifestyle preferences, our current generation of physicians has been mandated to limit the time they spend in residency training to eighty hours per week. This was based on evidence that mistakes were being made and learning suffered because of sleep deprivation. The new message to residents is that prolonged sleepless hours at the bedside are not good either for the patient or for the trainee. This message is a good one and will be taken forward. Even after the eighty-hour requirement, it is likely that these trainees will *appropriately* limit their hours in practice; they are telling us that they want more time to have a life outside of medicine, to be with their families. As a result, the next generation of physicians is expected to be ten percent less productive. And many are graying and will leave practice in the near future. A third of the nation's 750,000 physicians are over the age of fifty-five, which means that they probably will retire in ten to fifteen years. We are already seeing evidence of this trend: the most recent workforce study reported that current physicians say they are going to retire at two percent per year, twice the current rate, and other estimates suggest that by 2020, physicians will retire at a rate of 22,000 a year, up from 9,000 in 2000.

The take-home message on physician supply: the total number of hours worked by physicians (number of physicians times hours of work per physician) is likely to decrease from where we are today, despite an increasing demand.

DEMAND FOR PHYSICIANS: WHY WE NEED MORE

When it comes to trying to determine the appropriate number of physicians over the next twenty years, here are some inescapable facts.

Aging of the Population

In the United States today, thirteen percent, or approximately thirty-five million, of our population is aged sixty-five and older. In 2011, "Baby Boomers" will begin turning sixty-five. Ten thousand "Boomers" per day will then reach this milestone over the next twenty years and by 2030, the number of people aged sixty-five and older will have doubled to seventy-one million, representing one in five Americans. This aging will translate into much greater demand for medical services. One example of this is the expected forty-seven-percent increase in the demand for cataract surgery over the next fifteen years. In addition, the fastest-growing segment, those aged eighty-five and older, will rise in number from four million to twenty million by 2050, and will place the greatest demand upon the medical system.

Increased Burden of Chronic Illness

We are living longer with chronic disease; approximately forty-five percent of Americans have chronic disease, with eighty-eight percent of the population over sixty-five years old having at least one chronic disease, and twenty-three percent having five chronic diseases or more. This rising rate of chronic disease will also drive the need for more physicians because it takes time to treat patients with multiple chronic diseases. One recent estimate states that it would take 10.6 hours a day for physicians to provide all the recommended screenings and services to their chronically ill patients, more time than physicians have in a day to meet the medical care needs of *all* their patients, not just the half with chronic diseases. Therefore, combining the Baby Boomers, our insatiable demand for services ("right now"), our growing number of chronic illnesses, and our ability to treat chronic disease, demand for medical care is going to increase markedly: more need for physicians.

Advances in Medicine

Throughout decades and now centuries, medical science has delivered innovative therapies to improve medical care, and we can expect continued advances in medicine over the next ten years.

1. We will be better able to predict in *any individual* patient what diseases are likely to occur. We will then apply preventive treatment to those who are likely to benefit. The goal of better individualized strategies is to keep people alive and in the best possible health. But better health of the entire U.S. population is not likely to be realized in the next ten years. There will likely be a number of preventive strategies leading to increased monitoring (for example, more tests to be sure that the prevention is "working"), and so in the "near term" of ten years, we are not likely to need fewer physicians on this basis.

2. We will have the ability to determine *in the individual patient* which drugs will work best for an increasing number of diseases such as

infections and cancer. This type of personalized medicine will require more sophisticated testing and not less, leading to increased survival with chronic disease, and an increased need for care.

3. We will be able to prevent disease. A greater understanding of the human genome will give physicians the ability to identify people who are likely to get certain diseases and then to manipulate an individual's genes so she or he does not have the disease (either by destroying bad genes or inserting good genes). Although it may sound more like science fiction, this is science that we will start to realize in the next ten years. Initially, this will require *more* physicians to help guide the "genetic revolution" in terms of medical care and safeguarding patient privacy. Our doctors are not trained in the use of genetic therapy, and it is likely that this approach will be so advanced that there will be a need for new specialists in genetic therapy. The first attempts to solve single gene problems like hemophilia or cystic fibrosis are likely to involve intensive effort with ongoing monitoring and treatment, requiring more physicians. Eventually, perhaps twenty years from now, the "one-time fix" prevention of manipulating the genes and truly rendering the patient free of that disease will begin to occur, hopefully staying as healthy as possible until shortly before one's death, *then* leading to a reduced need for physicians.

4. Finally, we will have better technology, such as better images to show coronary heart disease and colon cancer without needing to put tubes into the body, and better instruments to do basic surgery (for example, replacing heart valves by threading tubes through the arteries and veins rather than opening the chest). The shifts in these types of procedures may change a bit what, for example, heart surgeons and cardiologists do, but these changes in technology are not likely to impact the overall need for physicians.

Waste

As we discussed in Chapter 3, we are probably providing too many services to patients, perhaps as much as twenty-five percent. By that reasoning, when we start doing the "right things" we should have more time and need fewer physicians. However, you may also recall from Chapter 3 that at present, half of all adult Americans do not receive many important medical services. Therefore, as we replace waste with more appropriate treatment, it is not likely that we will need fewer physicians.

The Uninsured

Within the next ten years, the United States will have to come to grips with the sixteen percent of the population that is uninsured. As we will see in Chapter 17, at best, the uninsured get about half of the care they need, and when they do have coverage, the need for physicians will increase.

Information Technology

Electronic medical records are truly likely to save physicians' time. At present, when a patient is seen, a paper chart—sometimes three to six inches thick—requires review. With electronic medical records, the time for this review can be shortened considerably and, on return visits, can include reminders to the physician and patient relating for necessary tests, which will improve care as well as save time. In addition, the administrative work of billing will be markedly reduced as notes from visits and procedures entered into the electronic record will be "understood" by a billing system and will be billed automatically. Tests and prescriptions will also be ordered automatically based on the information in the electronic medical record. There will be no need for letters to physicians who refer the patients, since, with appropriate password access provided by the patient, physicians who need to know about the patient have access to that record electronically. In today's world, electronic medical records are thought to save at best very little physician time, but there is evidence that electronic records do improve patient care. It has been estimated that in the next fifteen years, electronic medical records will save time and improve physician productivity by ten to thirty percent. If this is true, there could be an actual savings of perhaps fifteen percent in a physician's day. All things being equal, that would mean that the need for physicians might decrease by fifteen percent; however, it might also be that an individual physician who currently sees a large number of outpatients with an average visit of ten minutes might actually lengthen that visit by fifteen percent to eleven-and-a-half minutes. Time will tell.

Putting it all together in terms of the need for physicians as medicine changes over the next ten years, we have, at best, flat supply but with markedly increased demand. Increasing numbers of Baby Boomers, many with chronic disease, will turn sixty-five. As a result we can expect to see a marked increase in demand for medical care. Advances in medical care may require more physicians rather than fewer over the next ten years. Our best hope is information technology, perhaps improving efficiency and definitely improving the care of the patient. However, the improvement in efficiency is not likely to produce a real dent in the problem.

CAN WE FILL THE GAP FOR MORE PHYSICIANS?

What can we do? We can increase the number of medical students. Estimates are that we may need somewhere between 90,000 and 200,000 more physicians between now and 2020; and recent recommendations are to increase enrollment by thirty percent—or 5,000 new graduates per year—over the next ten years. Yet, even if medical schools *were* able to boost enrollment by thirty percent, the ratio of physicians to patients would still begin to decline by 2025. And, no matter how quickly we try to add new physicians we likely will still be lagging behind other developed countries. In fact, four of the countries below us in the OECD rankings (Australia, New Zealand, England, and Canada) are attempting to double their physician supply. This means that our rank of thirteen in the OECD countries for physician-to-population ratio could fall as low as seventeenth out of twenty in the near future.

In short, it doesn't appear that we will be able to meet the increased need for physicians in the near future. In a recent survey of deans of medical schools, some medical schools reported being able to increase class size an average of less than eight percent. This is because any larger increases in enrollment would require major facility changes (e.g., classrooms and laboratories) and an increase in the number of teachers. In addition, as the number of medical students increases, so will the number of residency positions need to increase. At present, funding provided by government for medical schools is mainly from the states, whereas for residency physicians, it is from the federal government. Even with the governmental support, many medical students begin their career deeply in debt, often owing more than $100,000 in loan repayments. This level of debt often persuades young people not to go into medicine in the first place, and those that do largely avoid practicing in rural areas or in medical specialties that have lower salaries.

To accomplish a real increase in physician supply in the United States, the federal government, the states, and the private sector will have to be involved in truly funding medical school and residency education so that debt is no longer an issue; some ideas that have been advanced: (a) creation of loan forgiveness programs for medical students; (b) free tuition for medical school; such tuition would cost the federal government less than half a billion dollars per year. At least some of these financial incentives could come with a requirement for intermediate-term two-to-five-year medical practice "placements" in medically needy areas (two to five years would allow them to become true members of the community) in return for the tuition support; (c) better wages for residents, who make about $10 per hour well after their thirtieth birthday, in poor comparison with their professional friends in other disciplines; and (d) subsidies to medical schools and teaching hospitals to increase their facilities and teaching faculties to handle the increased demand for students.

Finally, we will need to leverage the abilities of other outstanding practitioners such as nurses, nurse practitioners, physician assistants, and pharmacists to work at the maximum level of their licensure, or perhaps with more training, widen their licensure. For example, teams of generalists and specialists, each with a nurse practitioner, could care for patients with chronic disease such as congestive heart failure. The good news is that health professional education is moving toward collaborative training models; the bad news is that we already have a nursing and pharmacist shortage. It is hoped that with more and different types of job opportunities, these professions will become even more attractive and will increase their numbers.

The message is pretty clear: more Baby Boomers need more doctors. At some point in the near future, we will all hear that message.

⑫

MYTH: THE CURRENT MALPRACTICE SYSTEM HELPS PATIENTS

PROBLEMS WITH THE CURRENT MEDICAL MALPRACTICE SYSTEM

The current medical malpractice system is intended to help patients, censure doctors, and ultimately improve the quality of medical care; it does none of these terribly well.

Help patients? One goal is to help patients recover financially when a doctor injures them and is found to be negligent. The financial recovery of a medical malpractice lawsuit is intended to provide for:

1. Economic damages from loss of work—to pay the patient for estimated income they would have received had they not been injured;
2. Economic damages needed to pay for medical care expenses; and
3. Non-economic damages for things such as "pain and suffering," and loss of companionship.

The ideas sure seem reasonable, and occasionally, patients who are truly the victims of negligence are appropriately paid. The rules of estimating expenses do favor the patient. Most often, damages are based on the prediction that the person would have continued to work into the future; the likelihood of being laid off or demoted is not figured in; in fact, the person may collect the damages and continue to work. The person may also apply for disability from the U.S. government whether or not the patient has a private insurer who pays the bills (although not all states allow this type of double payment).

So what's the problem? For starters, when there *is* an award that is carefully justified and calculated, the patient goes home with only forty percent, because in many cases, sixty percent of every dollar awarded goes to attorney expenses (the major portion), with a smaller portion to administrative fees. It seems that attorney expenses and fees should be *additive* to the damages or else this makes a mockery of all of the "science" that went into calculating the damages. For example, if the patient is fifty-five years old and was making $75,000 and could not work, allowing for retirement at sixty-five, damages that might be awarded are $750,000 for missing the next ten years of work, with medical care expenses of $100,000 ($10,000 per year) plus $150,000 in non-economic damages for pain and suffering, for a total of $1 million. If the attorney takes $600,000, how is the person who cannot work going to pay her rent and other expenses that she was covering with her $75,000-per-year salary plus medical bills of $10,000 (total $85,000) when she only gets $40,000 a year from the award? In this example, it seems that if the attorney fee is to be $600,000, this should be added to the total award above and beyond what is awarded to the patient, for a total of $1.6 million. Attorneys should certainly be compensated at whatever level seems fair, but it would seem more reasonable to make this payment known and up front, rather than as a deduction from an award established in a rigorous fashion based on the type and level of the negligence. Having lawyers' fees as an add-on to the damages rather than as a deduction from the damages is already done in other types of litigation such as civil rights cases, and should be done as well in medical malpractice litigation.

DOES THE SYSTEM HELP INJURED PATIENTS?

Thus far, we have assumed malpractice actually occurred and the patient received an award. However, this is not always the case: only eight to thirteen percent of cases go to trial, and of those cases, the plaintiff (the patient) wins only about thirty percent of the time. Why? There are at least two possibilities:

1. Perhaps the judgments are correct, and there was in fact no malpractice the other seventy percent of the time. How we get the "right answer" to this, i.e., was there or was there not *really* malpractice, is difficult, because looking back at a case will still be done by different experts who may see the case differently.
2. The process of civil litigation is not perfect. Perhaps a true anecdote will add some light. A physician was found to be guilty of malpractice. In questioning the jury foreman after the award, the doctor's attorney was told that the jury "trusted the plaintiff's attorney because the attorney was born with one arm and must have worked very hard to overcome his handicap," and "the defendant doctor" who had been absent for three days of the ten-day trial to care for his patients, "must not have cared about this patient or he would have been here every day." Enough said.

So, since attorneys know that not many of their cases are likely to win, it is no surprise that attorneys are more and more likely to accept only those cases that are likely to bring large awards, which ensure the thirty-to fifty-percent fee needed to cover the expenses of other cases that they are going to lose and for which they get no payment. In our system, this implies that the low-income person with no health insurance who has a valid claim and simply wants to have their medical bills of $10,000 paid may not be able to find an attorney. So is this kind of medical malpractice system good for the patient?

DOES THE SYSTEM PREVENT FUTURE PHYSICIAN NEGLIGENCE?

Does the number of malpractice lawsuits brought against a physician identify a bad doctor? Not really: only seventeen percent of claims appear to involve a negligent injury. When a physician is sued, it is devastating for him or her, generally leading to self-doubt that may persist for years. In those cases where such doubting is healthy, this is a good thing, but to those who have tried their best, and, in fact, done nothing wrong despite a bad outcome, the malpractice process can be sufficiently traumatic to cause a physician to leave the profession. Does the system improve the quality of medical care? Remember the elements of quality from Chapter 9. Let's deal with safety, effectiveness, and efficiency.

Safety

Only about two percent of true medical errors ever result in malpractice claims. In other words, there are a large number of medical errors and avoidable injuries that occur that are never addressed within the malpractice system. It is not likely that safety will improve even if the number of malpractice claims doubled from two percent to four percent; ninety-six percent would still be unaddressed.

Effectiveness

As malpractice rates increase, physicians in certain specialties that handle higher-risk procedures, like obstetricians and neurosurgeons, are already leaving the practice of medicine and others are leaving the states with high malpractice rates. This creates substantial access problems for those needing care and is a real problem in rural regions, where some patients may have to drive 150 miles to see an obstetrician.

Efficiency

We spend about $7 billion a year on the direct cost of malpractice litigation. Surely this is too much by any other standard around the world. Also increasing the cost of medical care is the expense of doctors practicing "defensive medicine." Experts argue about the amount of money spent by doctors practicing defensive medicine, and in Chapter 3 we noted that practicing defensive medicine may account for as much as nine percent of health spending. Part of the difficulty in coming up with a number is in deciding what types of care are provided just to protect the physician. One study has concluded that it was not possible to tell from reading any medical record whether a physician ordered a test because of the fear of malpractice. So why not ask physicians whether they are practicing defensive medicine? In a recent survey, large numbers of doctors reported that they ordered more tests, referred more patients, prescribed more medication, and suggested surgical biopsies more often than was necessary because of concerns about malpractice. But in a second study, using hypothetical situations of medical care provided to patients, changing how one cared for patients because of a concern of being sued seldom exceeded five percent of all treatment decisions, which suggests that doctors may overestimate their use of defensive medicine. And even when doctors pointed to malpractice concerns as the most important reason to do a procedure, most of them also indicated other reasons such as "find a rare disease," or "to improve treatment," or even "patient's peace of mind." Therefore, asking physicians about their practice style may not provide reliable answers about how much the fear of malpractice drives them because, in most cases, they also believe what they are doing is the right thing to do for the patient.

In summary, defensive medicine is certainly practiced, but there is little evidence that doctors treat patients in certain ways *only* because of the fear of being sued.

TRYING TO FIX A BROKEN SYSTEM

The system doesn't work. Why? Part of the reason is that each part of it involves people who try to be objective but may not always be: the patient has been injured and is angry; the doctor is hurt, defensive and angry; the lawyer has a job to do; the jury may not understand the fine points of medicine and relies on which expert witness they believe, but all experts have their own bias. What to do?

1. Declare obvious malpractice before it goes to court. The listing of those issues in which malpractice occurs, such as taking off the wrong leg, can be settled quickly; other cases can be compared with national practice guidelines. For example, if a physician does something that is *not* indicated in a guideline and the physician does it anyway, and the patient is injured, this could be considered negligent and appropriate for a payment unless demonstrated that the guideline did not apply in

that particular case. Or, if a patient does not need a pacemaker (according to guidelines) and a physician implants one anyway—and the pacemaker becomes infected, causing a grave illness, this is negligence. In these cases, the physician would clearly need to apologize to the patient for the injury and the patient would receive payment according to a determined schedule of damages related to seriousness of the injury, the likely disability and some amount for non-economic damages ("pain and suffering"). The need for attorneys in these cases would be reduced.

2. "Health Courts" are an interesting idea where a judge (or a tribunal) who is experienced in malpractice decides the case rather than a jury. Experienced health care judges would work full time in these types of medical malpractice courts, and two or three non-biased experts paid by the court would testify to ensure all sides of the case were represented and to guard against any conflicts of interest.

3. Many states are trying to address the access, cost, and quality problems of the medical malpractice system. The vast majority of states have implemented: (a) a cap on non-economic damages because it is difficult to determine how to gauge pain and suffering. Some states have found a level of $250,000 to be sufficient, and have capped awards at that amount. Interestingly, it appears that the amount of overall awards in lawsuits in these states may not decrease since the cap on damages becomes the standard for what is demanded, rather than a lower number, which might have been the case before the cap was set; (b) regulations preventing "double recovery" of fees for medical care when a patient's insurance covers the care; and (c) proposing fee schedules for attorney's fees, much like for the vast majority of physicians.

We shouldn't need the legal system to determine whether a doctor is able to practice medicine. Physicians should review a physician's performance long before a lawsuit is threatened. As we discussed in Chapter 9, more outcome data are becoming available regarding physicians' quality performance, and so, fortunately, we increasingly have the opportunity to evaluate ourselves using national guidelines and standards. It may be a few more years until data are accurate enough at the level of the individual physician, but when the data are available, those physicians with borderline outcomes should be identified, whether by hospitals, health plans, or the state board of medicine. We must put into place programs that help those clinicians who are deficient to improve. And in those cases where the medical care remains of unacceptable quality, we must not permit that person to practice.

⓭

MYTH: MANAGING CARE IS EVIL

WHAT IS MANAGED CARE?

We have been talking about "managing care" throughout this entire book: addressing waste, using clinical practice guidelines to promote quality health care, and the importance of patient responsibility. There is nothing wrong with *managing* care. But managed care took on a special "Darth Vader" meaning in the 1990s, and that view remains.

Managed care has been defined as "influences in addition to the patient's physician that manage health care." The entire concept of managed care was wrapped up in the package of the health maintenance organization (HMO). The HMO is an insurance company that takes money in (from employers or individuals or even the government) and then contracts with health providers such as physicians and hospitals to pay for the medical care for patients. In the early days of managed care, HMOs had their own physicians who worked full time for that HMO. However, over time, the HMO began to contract with other physicians outside the HMO as well. The HMO originally had wonderful goals—to keep people well and to provide medical treatment when they became ill—which not only held the promise of better quality care but also the ability to control costs. Some of the techniques used by HMOs included:

1. Each enrollee in the health plan would be able to select his or her own primary care physician who always saw the patient whenever the patient needed medical treatment. This provided continuity in the patient's care because the physician knew the patient so well that the doctor could determine when a specialist was needed. This type of care coordination on the part of the primary care physician became known as the "gatekeeper" function since the primary care physician was determining whether to "open or keep the gate closed" to specialist physicians. Specialists provided important care when needed, but they were also much more expensive. Before managed care, patients often referred themselves to a specialist, whether their primary care physician thought it was a good idea or not. The entry of HMOs gave the role of specialty referral to the primary care physician, who, through their ongoing relationship with the patient, could better judge whether the patient needed the addition of specialized medical care.

2. The other major goal of the HMO was to save money. In the early 1990s, the United States was in an economic recession. Large corporations believed that the growing expense of employee health care benefits decreased companies' ability to compete in the world market. Lee Iacocca, then chairman of Chrysler, made his now-famous statement that his company "spent more on medical care than it did on steel for its cars." The HMO was seen as a possible "savior" to combat the spiraling increases in health care costs. Executives in large companies such as Chrysler had heard about the successes of HMOs (mostly on the West Coast) that were able to control costs better than other kinds of insurance companies. A major difference between HMOs and traditional insurance plans was the way they paid their physicians. In most insurance plans that were not HMOs, physicians were paid within a "fee-for-service" model, where every office visit and every operation was paid for separately as it was provided to the patient. Since physicians controlled how much was done, fee-for-service models allowed physicians to perform tests and provide other kinds of services and get paid whether or not the tests or services were

absolutely necessary. In an effort to reduce what the HMO thought might be unnecessary care, the HMOs decided to pay physicians in a different way called "capitation," in which physicians were paid a certain amount of money for each person under their care every month whether the physician saw the patient or not. This "capitation payment" had to cover whatever the patient needed, whether it was one office visit or expensive diagnostic testing or procedures. There were a number of capitation arrangements, but eventually the one that became most popular was one where the patient's primary care physician would receive the monthly amount of money from a patient's health plan for all physician care and some lab tests, and if the patient needed additional specialty care the primary care physician would have to pay, out of that initial monthly payment, the specialists to whom they referred the patient. This set up a direct financial conflict between different physicians caring for the same patient. Right or wrong, the HMOs were able to get physicians to go along with these payment arrangements since the HMOs "controlled" most of the patients: employers contracted with the HMO, and the HMO could say to physicians and hospitals, "take our deal or have no patients."

WHAT WENT WRONG?

Despite the original very reasonable goals (having a consistent primary care physician who coordinated medical treatment and eliminating wasteful practices that increased health care costs), HMOs became tarnished. Why?

1. Since the demands on primary care increased markedly, many physicians were booked months in advance, and patients were given appointments to see substitute physicians. The idea of having one's own physician who knew the patient well began to disappear as did the choice of physician, and, therefore, the first goal of managed care did not happen.
2. Capitation, originally conceived of as a way to reduce unnecessary care and limit services appropriately, also did not work as expected. Primary care physicians did limit testing and referrals to specialists, but in some

cases more than they should have, because they wanted to hold on to the monthly capitation payments in case a patient became seriously ill and required a great deal of resources. Since the payment came out of their own pockets, physicians were often put in the difficult position of either doing that extra test for a patient, or taking a salary cut. This conflict reflected the downside of managed care because just as there were positive incentives to keep patients well through preventive services and primary care, there were also negative incentives to withhold costly care even when needed. Physicians began to feel like "double agents," balancing the needs of patients against the needs of the patient's employer who wanted to spend less, or even against themselves because of the possible reductions in their own payments.

3. In the early to mid-1990s, the effects on the quality of care of these limitations were difficult to measure because data about what worked in medicine was scarce and clinical practice guidelines were less available. Therefore, in the absence of quality data, the HMO medical director (who decided what the HMO would pay for) mainly "managed" the cost of providing care. In financial terms, managed care worked: the price of health insurance markedly decreased. In 1993, at the time HMOs were just beginning to catch on, the rate of yearly growth of health insurance premiums reached 10.9 percent, but, three years later, in 1996, during their peak, the rate of growth had decreased to less than one percent.

WHAT HAPPENED? THE REVOLT AGAINST MANAGED CARE

The American public decided that the choice of their physician was important to them, more so than ever thought. Patients became angry when they found problems both in keeping their own primary care physician and in being limited in their ability to choose to see a specialist.

Managed care became more about managing "costs" than "care." Employers changed HMOs more frequently in order to continue to decrease their costs, and employees were forced to pay more to stay with their old HMO in order to keep their physician. In time, partly as the result of an improving economy with more jobs, employees and employers rebelled and the HMOs had to loosen their strict rules about referrals to certain specialists and services.

Although many claimed that quality of care suffered during the managed care era, the data are not clear. In a large study looking at HMO performance between 1997 and 2001 in cancer and heart disease treatment, sixteen HMOs had more favorable outcomes, sixteen had less favorable outcomes, and forty-one showed no clear difference. In another study, there was evidence that investor-owned, for-profit HMOs delivered lower quality of care as measured by rates of preventive services such as immunizations and mammography. The vast majority of studies were in agreement on one issue: despite the cost savings of HMOs, patients were less satisfied with what they considered to be the main tradeoff—the lack of access to their usual provider, difficulty in making appointments, or the need to travel longer distances. Physicians and patients interpreted these tradeoffs as problems in providing or receiving quality health care, which led to lower levels of satisfaction.

Jerome Kassirer, then editor of the *New England Journal of Medicine*, said it best: "It makes no sense to have a healthcare system in which the name of the game is to avoid caring for sick people." And apparently the American public agreed, because a decade after the "managed care revolution" stormed the United States, health policy experts declared that we had reached the "end of managed care." With fewer restrictions and more choices, and a growing quality movement that stressed disease management services and coordination of care, the price of health insurance—not surprisingly—rebounded back up to 11.2 percent in 2004.

HMOs still exist, but there are fewer of them, and most have changed their practices. "Preferred provider organizations" (PPOs) are much more common now, where physicians are allowed to practice as they see fit, for the most part, as long as their quality is high. In some plans, physician payments, usually in the form of bonuses, are tied to higher quality. Like it or not, most people respond to financial incentives, and physicians are no different. Large purchasers of health care (like the government and large employers) understand that money influences behavior and are hoping that linking financial rewards to higher quality of care (and not necessarily more care) will improve medical treatment and reduce unnecessary costly care.

Managing care to produce the best possible outcomes for the greatest number of people at the lowest possible cost should be the goal of medicine. This is not evil. The managed care of the 1990s that pitted physicians against patients in the name of cutting cost most definitely *was* evil.

IV

COVERAGE: THE MYTHS OF INSURANCE, UNDERINSURANCE, AND UNINSURANCE

(14)

MYTH: IN AMERICA, THERE IS A "SAFETY NET" OF GOVERNMENT PROGRAMS PROVIDING HEALTH CARE FOR THE POOR

HOLES IN THE HEALTH COVERAGE SAFETY NET

FACT: No matter how poor you are, if you are between nineteen and sixty-four years old, for all practical purposes, there is *no* guaranteed safety net for health care in the United States.

FACT: No matter how poor you are, if you are between nineteen and sixty-four years old, for all practical purposes, there is *no* guaranteed safety net for health care in the United States.

No, this is not a misprint. It is so important that we wanted you to see it twice.

Who are the uninsured in this country? About sixteen percent of our population, or forty-six million people, have no health insurance coverage. The size of that figure—forty-six million—is not a number we can easily understand. To put it in perspective, forty-six million is a lot greater than the population of Canada (thirty-two million); forty-six million is more than the number of Americans covered by Medicare; and, forty-six million is more than the total population of twenty-four of our states. If you add to the forty-six million the number of Americans who are uninsured for all or part of a year, the number is closer to sixty million. Over half of the uninsured make less than $20,000 per year and minorities are much more likely to be uninsured than white Americans: thirty-four percent are Hispanic, twenty-one percent are African American, thirteen percent are Caucasian, twenty-nine percent are American Indian or native Alaskan, eighteen percent are Asian or South Pacific Islander, and sixteen percent report two or more races.

In order to understand why we have so many uninsured people in our country, we first need to understand how health care coverage is provided in the United States. It is easiest to think of the large groups by age: almost all of those over sixty-five are covered by the public Medicare program, and those between the age of nineteen and sixty-four receive private health insurance coverage either as an employee benefit ("employer-based insurance" —sixty-two percent in 2004), or purchase health coverage as individuals (seven percent) for themselves and their families. There is essentially no guaranteed public program for those between the ages of nineteen and sixty-four unless you are pregnant, disabled, or a parent who makes so little money as to be essentially unemployed. Children under the age of nineteen may be covered by their parents' insurance through work, or if the child is from a poor family, can be covered by Medicaid. Because of our patchwork of coverage, nineteen percent of Americans between the age of nineteen and sixty-four are uninsured, as well as about twenty-five percent of children under the age of nineteen—a total of forty-six million Americans.

We will discuss employer-based insurance in Chapter 15, and for our purposes in this chapter, we will discuss the role of public health insurance in providing access and coverage to health services. There are four major government programs that provide health care coverage:

1. *Medicare*, covering approximately forty-two million people, was created in 1965 and covers virtually everyone over the age of sixty-five. Medicare also covers those who are blind, have chronic kidney disease, and are permanently disabled. Medicare is financed primarily through payroll taxes paid to the federal government by employers and employees, but the program is also funded through premiums paid by the individual. Medicare requires a deductible (the amount the individual has to pay before Medicare pays—for example, $912 per hospital stay) and co-insurance (the percent of the bill that the individual pays—for example, twenty percent for physician services) for

hospitalization and physician fees. Medicare has limits on what it will pay for in-patient hospital care, for nursing home care, and for home health care. Medicare offers coverage of outpatient prescription drugs, the cost of which is related to the senior's income. Because Medicare by itself covers less than half of beneficiaries' total health care services, many of those over sixty-five have some sort of supplemental insurance like retiree health benefits or "Medigap" coverage to pay for services like vision, dental, hearing, and other types of routine health care.

2. *Medicaid*, covering approximately fifty million people, was also passed in 1965 and provides health care coverage for poor people: low-income children, pregnant women, elderly, and disabled individuals. Medicaid is a shared program between the federal and state governments and receives funds from both. Depending upon the per-capita income of the state, the federal government pays between fifty and seventy-six percent of the overall costs of the Medicaid program. States with lower per-capita incomes receive a higher percent "share" from the federal government. There are two major Medicaid programs that cover the poor at both ends of the age spectrum: seventy-five percent of the Medicaid population is made up of low-income children and parents, while the remaining twenty-five percent consist of low-income seniors or persons with disabilities. Although enrollment in Medicaid has grown from four million in 1966 to over fifty million today, not everyone who is eligible enrolls in the program, often because it is neither easy nor convenient to enroll. Only seventy-two percent (twenty-five million) of eligible children and fifty-one percent (fourteen million) of eligible non-elderly adults are enrolled, suggesting that the ranks of Medicaid could grow by more than twenty million to a total of over seventy million if all the eligible children and non-elderly participated. For those who are over sixty-five years of age and poor (the so-called "dual eligibles"), Medicaid pays for Medicare premiums as well. Medicaid pays for more than sixty percent of nursing home residents. Medicaid provides coverage to persons with disabilities: sixteen percent of Medicaid beneficiaries are disabled and between the ages of nineteen and sixty-four. Medicaid pays for the first two years of disability before an individual is eligible for permanent disability coverage under Medicare.

The determination of "how poor" one needs to be to receive Medicaid coverage is set by the federal government and is related to the Federal Poverty Level (FPL), which is the way the United States measures poverty. The federal poverty guidelines were initially developed in the early 1960s based on the United States Department of Agriculture's definition of "nutritionally adequate diets for emergency use when funds are low": The department estimated that families of three or more people spent about one-third of their after-tax money on food, and then decided that three times the price of the "diet when funds are low" would become the Federal Poverty Level. The Federal Poverty Level has long been adjusted for inflation and family size since its introduction. It is no wonder that we have unusual multipliers like 133 percent, 200 percent, and 400 percent since the actual determination of the Federal Poverty Level was less than perfect from the start. But this imperfection remains: although the federal government has reviewed the way we measure poverty in the U.S. four different times since 1965, no changes have been made in the official poverty definition.

There were thirty-seven million people living below the poverty line in 2004, almost thirteen percent of the U.S. population, and the poor are disproportionately children (17.8 percent of all children) and black (24.7 percent of African Americans). By federal guidelines, Medicaid will cover pregnant women and children under the age of six whose family income is less than 133 percent of the FPL, as well as older children between the ages of six and nineteen living in families with incomes less than 100 percent of the FPL. The poverty line varies by size of the family. For example, a single mother with one child are considered poor in 2006 if their annual income is less than $13,200; for a family of four the FPL is $20,000. Therefore, Medicaid would cover pregnant women and children under six in a family of four if the family income was $26,600 (133 percent FPL) or less, and older children as well if the family's income fell below the poverty line of $20,000. Finally, Medicaid covers parents between the ages of nineteen and sixty-four who are extremely poor: their family income cannot exceed forty-one percent of the FPL, or $8,200 for a family of four. For all practical purposes, Medicaid does not cover working parents, and does not cover single adults between the ages of nineteen and sixty-four no matter how poor.

3. *The State Children's Health Insurance Program (SCHIP)* became available in 1997 and provides federal matching funds to help states expand health care coverage to the nation's uninsured children. SCHIP is administered by the states with each state setting its own guidelines regarding eligibility and services. The program covers almost four million children and "fills in coverage" for those children less than nineteen years of age whose parents make "too much" for Medicaid, but still fall below two-hundred percent of the Federal Poverty Level. Like Medicaid, it is paid for by the states and federal government, but the federal government's funding "match" is greater in SCHIP than in Medicaid. Although twenty-five million children are in Medicaid and four million more are covered by the SCHIP program, almost nine million children remain without health insurance coverage, with two out of three of them (6.2 million) eligible for either Medicaid or SCHIP.

States have the option in both Medicaid and SCHIP to increase the coverage beyond the federal minimums, and some states, like Tennessee, have elected to cover poor adults under Medicaid, while other states, like Arizona, have chosen to expand their SCHIP programs to cover parents and children. In most situations, when state budgets expand, Medicaid and SCHIP programs also expand their budgets and, alternately, when state budgets tighten, Medicaid and SCHIP services are reduced, leaving previously covered individuals without health insurance.

4. *The Veterans Administration (VA) program* covers approximately five million people who are retired from military service and their dependents. The Veterans Administration system provides medical, surgical, and rehabilitative care throughout 157 medical centers (with at least one in each state), and operates more than one thousand community-based outpatient clinics and nursing homes. The VA is the largest integrated health care system in the United States since it funds and provides health care.

WHY THERE ARE SO MANY UNINSURED DESPITE PUBLIC PROGRAMS

One might ask, "With all of these public programs, how can there be all of those uninsured people?" Here are some of the reasons.

1. Some of the uninsured are eligible for public health coverage but have not applied. Depending upon the state, as many as twenty-five percent of the children in families eligible for Medicaid or SCHIP do not apply. Why? Many say it is the regulations: some states have complex and lengthy applications that must be completed in person with proof that one lives in the state. In addition, proof of age, income, and assets with all the various documents like birth certificates, passports, tax forms, and wage slips, must be provided; applicants often are turned away if any of the information is missing. In some states, this procedure must be repeated every six months to "redetermine" eligibility. These types of administrative hurdles do little to increase enrollment, something we'll discuss further in Chapter 17. In addition to the administrative barriers, Medicaid's very low payment rates to physicians and other providers may reduce the number of providers willing to accept these rates, thus reducing access.

2. Each state has developed its own way of managing the needs of the uninsured, but many fall through the cracks. For example, most states have medical schools and teaching hospitals associated with state universities, such as the University of Virginia, that are charged as part of their mission with caring for the state's uninsured. Some states have county hospital systems like the Texas system of hospital districts. Unfortunately, in this type of system, if you do not live in the county with the hospital (even if you live in a bordering county), a person will not be covered by the county hospital and must travel to the state hospital. There are over 3,500 federally qualified community health centers (CHCs) throughout the country funded by the federal government. More than sixty percent of CHC patients are minorities, eighty-six percent earn less than 200 percent of the Federal Poverty Level, forty percent lack health insurance, and one-third speak a first language other than English. Despite the important role that they play in providing health care, these community health centers largely provide only primary care. With little access to specialists and limited geographic access, community health centers are only a partial solution in providing health services to the uninsured.

GETTING WORSE

The future looks no brighter: by 2013, the uninsured are estimated to grow to fifty-six million, representing almost one in five Americans, in part a result of the continued growth in health spending and the increasing cost of health insurance. Between now and 2013, health care inflation is estimated to be about eight percent per year whereas general inflation will be four percent. For every one percent that yearly inflation in health spending exceeds general inflation (and therefore wages) 246,000 people will lose health insurance, which means that between now and 2013, the number of uninsured Americans will increase by ten million.

Hubert Humphrey described the challenge we face today: "The true measure of society is in how it cares for those who cannot care for themselves: those in the dawn of life—the children; those in the twilight of life—the elderly; and those in the shadows of life—the sick, the needy, and the handicapped."

By this measure, our society has not done well.

15

MYTH: PEOPLE WHO WORK CAN AFFORD HEALTH INSURANCE

UNINSURED AND WORKING

The uninsured *do* work: they are the people you encounter every day who know your name, those who work at the cleaners, the restaurants, the gas stations, even in some department stores. More than eighty percent of the uninsured come from working families; almost seventy percent from families with one or more full-time workers. The number of the uninsured rose 800,000 between 2003 and 2004, and the great majority of the newly uninsured—750,000—were working adults between the ages of nineteen and sixty-four.

About fifty percent of working Americans are employed by small businesses with fewer than 200 employees, where only about fifty-nine percent of firms offer health insurance to their employees. Not surprisingly, the smaller the company, the less likely they are to offer health insurance. Only forty-seven percent of firms with three to nine workers offer health insurance, compared with ninety-three percent of businesses that have over 200 employees.

The future does not look promising. As a result of rising health insurance premiums—a seventy-three percent increase since 2000—employment-based health coverage continues to decline. In 1987, seventy percent of all U.S. businesses offered health coverage to workers, compared with sixty-nine percent

in 2000, sixty-six percent in 2003, and sixty percent in 2005. This is the lowest
level of employment-based insurance coverage in more than a decade. The
principal reason for the decline in employer-based health insurance coverage
is the continued erosion of employment-based insurance coverage in small
firms.

THE INSURANCE MARKET FOR INDIVIDUALS

For those whose employer does not offer insurance, the only way they can
obtain health coverage is in the "individual insurance market" where they
go to an independent insurance broker and directly buy an insurance plan
for themselves or their family, just like automobile insurance. The individual health insurance market is the only source of health insurance for the
more than one out of five Americans who are not eligible for group or public health insurance. About seventeen million persons, about seven percent
of those under sixty-five, purchase individual health insurance each year.
Individual insurance premiums vary more than group premiums paid by
large businesses, and generally the benefits are less generous. The price can
vary from less than $1,000 per year for coverage for a single person to over
$8,000 for family coverage, with average premiums of $2,531 for a single
person and $4,442 for a family.

In order to understand how working Americans deal with the individual
health insurance market, let's assume a family of four where the parents are
in their mid-thirties and no one in the family has had any unusual health care
expenses. For this type of family, an average health insurance premium would
be $4,000 with a $1,500 deductible (the amount the person has to pay out of
pocket before insurance starts to pay). Let's also assume that both parents
work in a local small business, such as a restaurant or dry cleaners, and are
paid minimum wage at $5.15 per hour, making a combined income of
$21,424 per year. Remember from Chapter 14 that the Federal Poverty Level
for a family of four is $20,000. Therefore, the family makes too much even for
the two children to be covered by Medicaid. So, they are on their own to pay,
at a minimum, $5,500 in premiums and deductibles, when they bring home
only $21,424 before taxes; that's over twenty-five percent of their income.

What if they had employer-sponsored health insurance? For small and
large firms, average annual premiums are fairly similar, with smaller firms'

premiums about eighteen percent higher than premiums in larger firms for equivalent benefits. As mentioned in the first part of this chapter, smaller firms are much less likely to offer health insurance. When they do offer access to a health plan, workers in small firms pay significantly more of their money for family coverage—in terms of percent of premium and in terms of deductibles—than workers in large firms. We explore the reasons for this in Chapter 16. The average small business group-based premium for a family with two children is $10,880, with an average of $7,710 paid by the employer, leaving $3,170 paid by the employee. Finally, if we then take the "best of all worlds," the same family working for a large employer, the same average annual premium of $10,880 would apply, but this time the business covers over three quarters of the premium and passes along $2,487, or twenty-three percent of the premium, to the employee. Therefore, we see that for our low-income family in the individual market (with no employer to pay anything), the premium would be thirty percent of income; for the same family covered through a small business it would be approximately fifteen percent of income; and if the family received coverage through a large business, twelve percent of income. Yet even this comparison across the three different health insurance markets is only part of the story: average deductibles are higher for workers in small businesses, often as much as $200 per year higher than the average of $300–$600—and benefits are also generally less generous (for example, often there is less coverage for prescription drugs or access to specialists) when purchased as an individual plan.

The cost of the premium also depends upon the age, gender, health status of the individual or family, and the amount of the deductible (as described in Chapter 10). In general, older purchasers pay higher premiums than younger purchasers, reflecting the greater risk of getting sick as one gets older. Premiums also vary, depending upon how healthy the person is, or for example, whether coverage for pregnancy and newborn care are desired. In one state, a healthy twenty-five-year-old male could purchase a policy with coverage for prescription drugs and mental health benefits and a $2,500 deductible for $625 per year, while the same policy for a healthy sixty-three-year-old man is almost $3,000. If the sixty-three-year-old was deemed "unhealthy," a similar insurance plan, assuming it was available (and often it is not) would cost $10,800. It is no wonder then that nearly two-thirds of those seven million Americans who are individually insured tend to be in excellent health; unfortunately, for those who are sick who need coverage the most, the premiums are too high.

HOW MUCH CAN PEOPLE AFFORD?

What is "reasonable" to expect an individual to pay as a percent of income? In surveys of those living in poverty, most say they would pay up to five percent of income for health care coverage. Health care is only one of many expenses in a household. For the average low-income family, thirty-three percent of their income is paid for housing, twenty percent for transportation, twenty percent for child care, seventeen percent for food, eight percent for clothing, and the remaining two percent for everything else. When you do the math less than $400 is what is left for health care if you make $20,000 per year. This is why most poor and low-income families report that they live "paycheck to paycheck" and decide which bills they can pay each month and delay the others; they shop at thrift stores, and use less expensive unlicensed child day care services in order to get by. Interestingly, operating a car costs about $8,000 per year—the same as a family health insurance premium in the individual market. If the car is absolutely necessary to get to work, they go without health insurance. Now it should be clear why most of the uninsured do not have health care coverage: they cannot afford it. Like our family above, thirty-five percent of the uninsured live in families with annual incomes of less than $20,000, and fifty percent live in families that make less than $25,000 per year.

For a family of four that receives employer-sponsored health care from a small employer and pays thirty percent of the $10,880 annual premium ($3,264), if the family makes less than $65,000, they are paying more than five percent of their income. As it happens, many American families do stretch their budgets and pay more than five percent of income. These are the people who are called the "underinsured," those who do have health insurance but have annual medical expenses that exceed five or even ten percent of income.

They are called "underinsured" because once the ten percent threshold of income is met, they are less able to pay for other out-of-pocket health expenses, such as co-insurance for doctor visits and prescription drugs—or less able to pay for the other essentials of daily life. The underinsured are almost as likely as the uninsured to delay needed medical care and to have medical debt. In a recent survey of the underinsured done by the Commonwealth Fund, more than one-third reported problems or delays in getting medical care because of the cost, and nearly two-thirds said they had trouble paying medical bills even though they had health insurance at the time of care.

However, there are eleven million people—twenty-five percent of the uninsured—who probably CAN afford health insurance coverage, with family incomes over $50,000 (after all, the same family plan in the individual market used for our low-income family would amount to less than ten percent of income). Perhaps these families prefer to pay out of pocket each time they need heath care, but what happens if they have a "catastrophic" medical event like cancer or an automobile accident? States are getting the idea: Maryland has proposed a tax penalty if individuals with incomes over $63,000 (four-hundred percent of the Federal Poverty Level) do not have health insurance, and Massachusetts' recent health reform plan includes a penalty for citizens who do not have health coverage.

HEALTH OR TELEVISION?

An estimated sixteen million people are underinsured in the United States. When added to the forty-six million Americans who have no health coverage, a total of sixty-two million, more than twenty percent of our population, are either underinsured or uninsured.

Remember this: The vast majority of the uninsured and the underinsured are low-income workers who cannot afford adequate health insurance. The decline in employer-based health coverage, particularly in small firms, combined with the growth in the mobility of the American workforce, may create a greater demand for the purchase of individual health insurance. Although individual coverage is relatively affordable for those who want to insure against only catastrophic medical accidents, it often is available only for those who are fairly healthy. Therefore, unless public policies are developed to balance affordability with availability for those other than the healthy, the individual insurance market will not be effective in expanding health coverage overall.

So the next time you hear somebody say, "You know everybody has a choice—they can either buy health insurance or televisions," tell them they don't know the half of it.

16

MYTH: PROVISION OF HEALTH INSURANCE FOR EMPLOYEES HAS ALWAYS BEEN THE EMPLOYER'S RESPONSIBILITY, AND WILL CONTINUE THAT WAY

A QUIRK OF HISTORY

Neither long tradition nor well-thought-out public policy is responsible for the fact that health insurance is arranged at the workplace through employers (so-called "employer-based" insurance). The practice came about during the wage freezes of World War II when employers were not permitted to attract scarce workers by increasing wages, but were allowed to provide free health care to employees and families as a benefit. The law was written such that health insurance was a "before-tax" business expense. Congress eventually added this benefit to the Internal Revenue Code and made permanent the status of employer-provided health insurance as a pretax benefit. Over time, providing employer-sponsored health benefits became "the way we do business."

PROS AND CONS OF THE EMPLOYER-BASED SYSTEM

Pros

Some of the positive reasons to maintain our uniquely American system of employer-based health coverage include:

1. *It works.* It has been there for as long as most employees can remember, most people like the way the system is arranged, and most workers in surveys say that they want their employer to continue providing health care as an employee benefit. In a survey that asked employees how they wished to receive health coverage, more than half replied that they preferred employment-based health care to government coverage or other coverage. Receiving health insurance at work is easy for the employee. The employer simply deducts the employee's share of the health insurance premium as part of the payroll process. This "automatic" payroll feature of the employer-based insurance system is attractive to employees. In fact, when asked if they would rather have their employer arrange for insurance or be given money to purchase it on their own, almost two out of three employees said they would rather have the employer arrange the insurance.

2. *It supplies a tax benefit to the employer* because it is considered a business expense and thus reduces the total cost of the health insurance. Take this example: if we assume a $6,000 health insurance premium with the employer paying seventy percent, the employer's cost for their employees' health insurance coverage is $4,200. But, because health insurance counts as a business expense, the company is taxed on an income that deducts the value of the health insurance business expense. Assuming the employer is in the twenty-seven-percent tax bracket, there will be a tax savings of twenty-seven percent of the $4,200 premium, which equals a savings of $1,134. As well, there are additional savings in Social Security, Medicare, and state taxes because they too will be taken out of the lower income, resulting in further savings of $531. After we add up the savings from the health insurance premium ($1,134) and the savings from the other taxes ($531) a total employer cost for his employee's insurance coverage is $2,535, a forty-percent savings overall. Now let's deal with the thirty percent

of the premium the employee has to pay: $1,800 of the $6,000 premium—but since employees also get to pay their part with "pre-tax" dollars, the employee in the twenty-five percent tax bracket saves $450. Overall, in using pre-tax dollars, the $6,000 premium costs $3,885. If this tax incentive were eliminated and the employer gave the employee the $2,535 (which is the amount of money truly spent), to buy the same insurance, the employee would have to spend $3,465 instead of $1,350. This type of savings through tax benefits provides incentives for the employer and the employee to have employer-based health insurance.

Cons

However, despite the tax and administrative advantages, employer-based insurance has some negative features, including:

1. *The problem of "job lock"*—a condition in which individuals have health insurance but feel "locked" into their present position for fear of losing health insurance coverage if they change jobs. This is a real problem for anyone who has a health condition because many insurance plans carry within their policies a "preexisting condition exclusion" where they exclude coverage for certain medical problems (such as cancer). If an employee has been insured through one employer for longer than a year and has therefore satisfied one insurance plan's preexisting condition exclusion, they will not want to face another waiting period by changing jobs and facing a year without coverage. This is true particularly for employees with chronic diseases and who are under active treatment (e.g., cancer chemotherapy). Recent laws have made preexisting condition exclusions illegal if the patient has had coverage for at least twelve months in a prior employer's health plan before moving to a new company's insurance plan. Unfortunately, these laws do not regulate the cost of the new insurance plan, and so those with preexisting conditions who change jobs may face extremely high premiums as they move from one job to another.

2. *The high administrative cost to business for arranging health care* in time and money. Health insurance was the largest employer-provided benefit in 2004, accounting for almost a third of all benefits. Many

employers, think the "hassle" of offering health insurance, which requires hiring internal benefits managers or expensive outside contracting agents, is too costly. In addition to the time investment, the administrative costs for billing and enrollment are also significant, particularly for small businesses, where insurance "loading charges" are built into the premiums, making them more expensive.

3. *For virtually all businesses (e.g., auto manufacturers) providing health care is not their "core business,"* yet they find themselves having to learn how to negotiate effectively with the health insurance industry in order to obtain the best price in quality health care. There is no question that purchasing health coverage for employees is an important business decision: over the past twenty years, employer health care costs have doubled as a percentage of average wages from 5.5 percent in 1984 to 11.6 percent in 2004. One positive aspect is that it provides them with opportunities to act as careful purchasers of health care. For example, the Leapfrog Group, a collection of more than 170 employer organizations that purchase health care for more than thirty-seven million people in the United States, has provided important leadership in using the employer-based health insurance system to require certain quality standards, based on national guidelines for physicians and hospitals. For example, they have insisted that hospitals provide round-the-clock coverage of intensive care units by physicians, and that hospitals use computers to reduce medication order errors. While the Leapfrog Group's efforts have been helpful in advancing the delivery of quality health care, the fact is, defining quality of medical care should be the job of the medical profession. Hopefully, as quality reporting improves and becomes more system-wide, we will take the lead and businesses will find it less necessary to "force" health practitioners to develop certain quality measures; in the long run, businesses should be informed buyers and hold providers accountable—but not create the metrics.

NOT ALL BUSINESSES ARE EQUAL

Large employers have made employer-based insurance routine, with ninety-eight percent of those with greater than 200 employees offering health insurance. Not so for small employers, who employ over thirty percent of the private sector workforce; only fifty-nine percent of those with fewer than two-hundred employees offer health care coverage. This is largely because of the smaller number of employees and the administrative complexity and expense for small business. Small businesses expenses are higher for a number of reasons:

1. *Administrative costs* to the insurance company to market and service small businesses may be up to forty percent greater than for large businesses. Small businesses are more likely than large firms to be in the goods and services labor sectors such as construction, restaurants, agriculture, and fishing. These labor sectors report higher percentages of employees that work part-time, have less education, and are on public assistance. There is much higher turnover with employees in small business, which requires more frequent changes in the updating of employee information, which, in turn, increases costs for the company.

2. *Those in small business generally have a higher risk of being injured.* Three-quarters of work-related injuries occur in the goods and services industries, such as restaurants and other small businesses, thus making health care costs and premiums higher.

3. *Expenses are higher for small businesses because there are fewer employees who can "share the risk."* For example, if one person in the company becomes extremely ill and runs up a large hospital bill, spreading the cost over an eight-employee pool is a lot more expensive than spreading it over a pool of eight hundred employees.

4. *There is a greater risk of adverse selection in small employer groups.* Because health insurance is more expensive for employers and workers in small businesses, the workers who do purchase insurance may do so because they have greater health needs, leading to what is known in the insurance industry as "adverse selection." This important concept of insurance directly relates to the ability to spread risk over a large number of employees. If only those who are sick buy insurance, this "adverse selection" increases the cost of the premium because there are fewer well people to pay for the costs of the sick members. In this way, the primary "insurance function" disappears, and very few well people sign up—meaning that the sick end up

paying for themselves through a very expensive, and often unaffordable, health insurance premium.

5. *A single small business with few employees has less "clout"* to negotiate health insurance premium rates compared to a large business. Because of the higher expense, a small business is able to offer less
choice of plans. In 2003, seventy percent of businesses with fewer
than 200 employees offered just one plan compared with eighty percent of large businesses that offered at least two choices. Having less
choice in plans, including the unavailability of a lower cost alternative,
means that young, healthy, or low-income workers may find the single
option employer-sponsored coverage too costly, and may choose not
to buy coverage at all.

Therefore, if small businesses provide health insurance at all, it is less
generous coverage than large businesses provide, because of greater administrative costs and the inability to spread risk, and because the products
they are offered by carriers are less affordable because of adverse selection.

Over the last five years, health insurance premiums have grown by
seventy-three percent compared with general inflation of fourteen percent
and wage growth of fifteen percent. If health insurance premiums continue
to grow, declining employer-based health insurance may become evident in
large businesses as well as small businesses. We will discuss this in more detail in Chapter 20.

While employer-based health care has no real historical basis in public policy except through the Internal Revenue Code, employer-based health insurance provides the majority of U.S. workers with coverage for health care and
protection from financial losses because of illness; compared with the individual market, it provides administrative efficiencies, insurance purchasing
clout to get the best prices and quality, and tax-advantaged funding. For all of
these reasons, and because it has worked for over a half century and continues to be very popular with employees, employer-based health insurance, in
some form, will likely continue to provide insurance for the majority of American workers—unless and until there is a major overhaul in the system.

17

MYTH: THE UNINSURED GET THE CARE THEY NEED IN EMERGENCY ROOMS

A MATTER OF LIFE OR DEATH

The truth of the matter is that the uninsured die earlier than the insured. Adults without health insurance have death rates twenty-five percent higher than insured persons. Generally speaking, the uninsured are at greater risk for premature death because they receive fewer preventive services and less effective treatment for acute medical conditions such as a heart attack. They are less likely to be admitted to a hospital, are less likely to receive treatments, and are more likely to die in the short term. The uninsured with chronic conditions, such as diabetes, high blood pressure, heart disease, and cancer, are sicker and die at a younger age largely because of delayed diagnosis and treatment. More than half of uninsured adults with diabetes go without needed medical care or prescription drugs each year, which puts them at increased risk of hospitalization for complications such as heart and kidney disease, amputations, and blindness. The uninsured with breast cancer and colon cancer have a thirty- to fifty-percent higher chance of dying from their disease than those with private insurance. The uninsured are also three times more likely than those with health coverage to postpone needed care for pregnancy, for injuries, or for cancer care, so it should come as no surprise that having health insurance improves health overall and reduces mortality rates by twenty-five percent. When you consider the benefits of having health insurance and access to needed medical care, it is clear that the uninsured do not get enough care.

HOLES IN THE SAFETY NET

What does our health care system do for America's uninsured? The uninsured are half as likely to receive needed care as those with health insurance; when they are sick, the uninsured seek medical care thirty-seven percent of the time, while the insured will seek care eighty-two percent of the time.

This is particularly troubling since nearly half (forty-five percent) of uninsured adults report having one or more chronic health conditions such as diabetes, cancer, high blood pressure, or heart failure, so they certainly require treatment. However, one-fourth of uninsured adults with chronic conditions report *no* doctor visits in the last twelve months, and half report skipping needed medical care or not filling a prescription because of the cost. Uninsured adults with chronic conditions were 4.5 times as likely to go without needed care as those with health coverage. Three out of five uninsured adults with chronic conditions received no dental care in the last year despite the fact that forty percent reported a need for the dental care.

Part of the reason many of the uninsured postpone or go without needed care is because over forty percent do not have a regular doctor's office to go to when they are sick, compared with less than ten percent of those with health coverage. Where *do* the uninsured get medical care? They go to emergency rooms. In fact, for one out of four uninsured patients, the emergency room is their only regular place of care.

Emergency departments have become the "family doctor" for America's uninsured, because emergency rooms are *required* to see all comers because of an unintended consequence of federal legislation. In 1986, Congress passed the Emergency Medical Treatment and Active Labor Act, which provides that any individual, regardless of their insurance status or ability to pay, who goes to an emergency room must be examined and initially treated (if need be) before being transferred to a different hospital. This legislation was intended to prevent the practice known as "patient dumping," in which a patient who had a true emergency (such as an automobile accident, a heart attack, or was about to give birth) was taken to a hospital emergency room, only to be transferred once it was learned that the patient had no health insurance or ability to pay. Patients were put into an ambulance and "dumped" at another hospital that was known to provide care for indigent patients, generally a public hospital or a hospital affiliated with a medical school. The uninsured quickly figured out that the law required the emergency room to treat them whether or not there was a true emergency, and so they began to use the emergency room for all kinds of medical treatment.

Emergency rooms are the usual source of care for increasing numbers of uninsured patients with emergency and non-emergency medical problems. But this safety net carries a price: emergency physicians and other specialists combined lose more than $4.2 billion in revenue each year as a result of providing the mandated care. Additionally, hospitals are paying $600 million a year to ensure that on-call specialty physicians are available in the emergency room setting, and still some communities cannot meet the demand.

If that isn't bad enough, emergency rooms are also experiencing severe overcrowding. In 2003, nearly 114 million visits were made to hospital emergency rooms, more than one for every three people living in the United States. Of the sixteen-plus million patients that arrived at emergency rooms by ambulance in 2003, 501,000 ambulances, or one per minute, were diverted because of emergency room overcrowding and lack of beds. And, once in the emergency room, patients sometimes wait up to two days to be admitted to an available hospital bed. How can this be? It is simply a case of supply and demand: In the last decade the population of the U.S. grew by twelve percent, hospital admissions increased by thirteen percent, and the number of emergency room visits increased by twenty-six percent. Despite this increased volume, the number of hospital emergency rooms *decreased* by twelve percent, mainly the result of hospital closings in response to lower reimbursements by managed care, Medicare, and other payors. By 2001, sixty percent of hospitals were operating at or over capacity. For uninsured patients, the reduced supply of emergency rooms has resulted in further restricting access to timely medical care.

The uninsured make eighteen million visits each year to the emergency room, almost seventeen percent of all visits. Eighteen million visits per year sounds like a lot, but it averages to less than one visit per person per year, as there are forty-six million uninsured in the United States. And, since we know that the uninsured use the emergency room as their clinic, this means that the uninsured are seeking medical care a lot less than the national average of about seven clinic visits per person per year for those with health insurance. In addition, as anyone who has visited an emergency room knows, these are not places to go for comprehensive medical care. Emergency rooms are designed to treat the "emergency" medical problems facing the patient who shows up for needed care, but emergency rooms do not typically address the underlying chronic disease or condition that may have contributed to the immediate problem. In truth, preventive care almost never happens in an emergency room. This is why those without health insurance are fifty percent less likely to have had preventive services such as pap smears, mammograms, and prostate exams compared with insured adults. It would make sense for physicians in the emergency room to refer their uninsured patients to an outside doctor's office or clinic for follow-up and preventive care, and they probably do, but the uninsured usually do not get follow up. Why? The reason is, in part, because doctors' offices and clinics are not required by law to see uninsured patients. And so it is no surprise that emergency room physicians report that finding specialists to accept referrals, and having the patient fill their prescriptions, are their toughest challenges in caring for uninsured patients, mainly because an increasing number of physicians are refusing to accept uninsured patients.

GOING WITHOUT HEALTH CARE IS EXPENSIVE TOO

Even with half the visits than those with health coverage, uninsured adults face large out-of-pocket expenses for their care. One in five, or twenty percent of those uninsured with chronic illnesses, spend at least $2,000 out of pocket. The uninsured are three times as likely to be contacted by a collection agency for non-payment of medical bills. This lack of care combined with medical bills becomes a vicious circle for the uninsured: more with illness → more miss work → less ability to pay → more uninsured → more illness. When this happens, we all lose, in individual health status and in productivity of our society. One of the reasons we have such disparities in health care among Hispanics, African Americans, the poor, and those living in rural counties and inner cities is because so many are uninsured and often have poorer health. Emergency rooms, charitable physicians, community health clinics, and other safety net providers, while helpful, cannot fully substitute for adequate health coverage. Remember what we said in the beginning of this chapter: researchers estimate that a reduction in mortality of twenty-five percent could be achieved if the uninsured had health care coverage.

No wonder our life expectancy is so low.

Martin Luther King Jr. put it best: "Of all the forms of inequality, injustice in health care is the most shocking and inhumane."

18

MYTH: NO ADDITIONAL FUNDING IS NEEDED TO COVER THE UNINSURED; THE MONEY IS AVAILABLE IN THE SYSTEM

While it may be true that there is plenty of money in the U.S. health system, the question becomes, can we actually get our hands on any of it to pay for the uninsured—in other words, is the money "available?" How much money do we need, what is the cost of care for the uninsured, and what do we currently spend?

WHAT DO WE SPEND NOW?

The uninsured receive a little more than half of the medical care per person compared with those who have health insurance, and total spending from all sources on medical care for the uninsured is around $125 billion. Many people think that those without health insurance in this country get "free care," but in truth, over a third (thirty-five percent) of the costs of care received by the uninsured are paid for by themselves as out-of-pocket payments. The other two-thirds of the costs are paid through public and private sources.

Almost sixty million people lack health coverage for all or part of a year, and of the $125 billion in medical care expenditures for the uninsured, having partial health insurance coverage through the year pays for $51 billion of the $125 billion. Most of the remaining costs are referred to as "uncompensated care costs," which comes to about $41 billion a year. This $41 billion in uncompensated care is funded by state and federal government programs that go toward payments to hospitals or community health centers to make up for financial losses they have when a large portion of their patients cannot pay their medical bills, by private dollars from higher health insurance premiums, and from true charity care. Doctors and clinics provide $6 billion in uncompensated charity care, with doctors providing the lion's share of truly "free care" that is not reimbursed at $5 billion.

How private insurance dollars directly and indirectly fund the uninsured is complex because of the hidden subsidies in private insurance that we all pay, although recent studies suggest that as much as $29 billion of private health insurance premiums may be used to help pay for medical care for the uninsured. This means that private insurance premiums are significantly higher than they would be if everyone had health insurance. These higher premiums pay for the unpaid care given to the uninsured and create a way that hospitals and doctors can receive some payment for the care they provide to the uninsured. This "cost shift" amounts to an average increase of 8.5 percent tacked on to everyone's private health insurance premium: $922 for every family policy and $314 for individuals, which brings in $29 billion per year to help pay for the uncompensated care of the uninsured. This is not done explicitly; it is simply negotiated among private insurers, hospitals, and physician groups who must find ways to reduce the financial losses incurred from treating the uninsured. Remember, clinics and doctors already provide over $6 billion of truly "free care" each year for the care of the uninsured. If the clinics and doctors are less successful in negotiating these higher rates with insurers, either the cost of totally free care they give will increase, or they may find themselves unable or unwilling to care for the uninsured at all because of the increased costs to them and their practices.

WHAT WILL IT COST?

The relevant question then becomes just how much more will it cost, over and above what is already being spent on the cost of medical care for the uninsured, to provide insurance coverage for those who do not have it?

Recently, estimates have been made of what it would cost to cover the uninsured. As we discussed above, the uninsured receive about half of the medical care per person compared with those who have insurance. According to experts, if all the uninsured, those who were uninsured all year as well as those who were uninsured for part of the year, gained health coverage, total yearly spending on medical services would increase by $48 billion. When added to the current spending level of $125 billion, the increase of $48 billion brings the total to $173 billion needed each year to provide health coverage for the currently uninsured. When viewed from a "macro" level, this new $48 billion investment, relative to current government spending for public health insurance programs, is quite small. Medicare and Medicaid alone *each* cost around $300 billion per year. The new dollars needed to offer the uninsured health coverage would constitute less than three percent of total personal health spending in the United States and would increase the current share of gross domestic product going to health care by less than one percent.

HOW MUCH MORE DO WE NEED?

How can we find the additional money, and how much do we really need? In order to lower their insurance premiums, would those with private insurance be willing to trade the $29 billion they currently pay in higher insurance premiums for an explicit tax to cover the uninsured? There are about 120 million individuals and families paying taxes, this would be $250 for every taxpayer, a figure close to the average of $314 that insured individuals now pay to cover the uninsured through the cross subsidy of their private insurance premiums. Clearly, as a tax, this new payment would likely be related to income, so each family would not pay the same amount; those who make more would pay a little more, and those whose income is less would pay less. But, if the public does not want to pay a new tax, even in exchange for lower premiums, and, over time, doctors and hospitals are no longer able to negotiate the higher rates to offset their charity care, there will be an even greater need to find *new* funding to pay for the care of the uninsured.

Assuming the public does not want to pay a tax of $29 billion needed to make up the loss of the higher premium payments, we have to add the

$6 billion in free care currently provided by doctors and hospitals—which they would no longer do if everyone was insured. This brings the total to $35 billion in new funds needed to cover uncompensated care, and, adding this figure to the $48 billion that would be necessary to provide full-year health coverage to all of the uninsured, we end up with having to find $83 billion in new funds.

WHERE CAN WE FIND THE MONEY?

So, can we find the $83 billion of "new money"? Where should we look? Let's start with the "waste" in our health care system; conservatively, there must be at least five percent that we waste (as we discussed in Chapter 3, most experts think it is a lot more). Five percent of $1.6 trillion is $80 billion; that's almost all we need. But as we discovered in Chapter 5, it is at least as likely that this waste will be counterbalanced by the added expense of providing higher quality care for those who are currently not receiving it. Therefore, while clearly cutting all waste out of the system is a worthy goal and should be part of any reform of the U.S. health care system, so should be providing higher quality care. Improving quality is likely to take up any dollars that we gain from cutting waste. As we said in Chapter 5, quality health care is not cheap.

Secondly, we might ask whether providing health insurance would improve productivity in the workforce, and if so, could we find new dollars there to pay for the coverage for the uninsured. It has been estimated that health insurance will decrease absenteeism and increase productivity by ten percent. This productivity linked to better health status is called "health capital." It is estimated that the value of the "health capital" that would be gained as a result of insuring all Americans equals $65 billion to $130 billion per year for society as a whole. This money would, theoretically, be available for paying for the uninsured, but businesses are more likely to find other ways to "reinvest" any such gains, such as increasing dividends to shareholders.

Thirdly, billing and other administrative costs very likely will decrease with the use of electronic medical records and electronic billing, a possible source of new funds. Reducing billing costs and other administrative efficiencies could save $60 billion a year. We know that public health program insurers like Medicare and Medicaid have administrative costs that are under five percent, much lower than the fourteen percent administrative costs found in private insurance. However, Medicare and Medicaid are huge programs with the ability to spread fixed costs over a very large population, and it is unlikely that private insurance, even with administrative efficiencies, could match the public programs' lower level of administrative costs. But perhaps we could shoot for something between five and fourteen percent, something around nine percent for administrative costs (a thirty-six-percent reduction). Billing costs are eight to twelve percent for hospitals and physician groups, so reducing administrative costs to an average of nine percent for all payers and providers (other than public) could bring significant savings and free up billions in new money, perhaps as much as $100 billion since it has been estimated that reducing our administrative spending to Canadian levels (roughly equivalent to Medicare) would save $140 billion annually. Again, the question is whether this potentially new revenue is "available" to help cover the uninsured. And, once again, the answer is probably not. Insurance companies and physician groups report that new information management costs (for example, in electronic health records) will exceed any future savings, at least over the next ten years. Therefore, as in our example of improved productivity, health care organizations and physician groups are *not* likely to consider these dollars "available" any time in the near future for the uninsured.

A fourth potential source of revenue is the "tax break" to employers. This tax treatment goes back more than fifty years, allowing for the purchase of health insurance with pre-tax dollars, discussed in Chapter 17. This tax subsidy was calculated at over $188 billion in 2004. With a single act, removal of this tax exemption could clearly solve the problem of paying for the care of the uninsured, since these dollars would now be collected by the federal government as taxes and could be used to provide direct subsidies for health coverage either through the public or the private systems. However, this too is unlikely: even though the employer-based insurance system is considered by many to be inefficient and unjust, it nonetheless will be difficult to change, as we discussed in Chapter 16 and will revisit in Chapter 19.

Finally, what about the rollback of the Bush tax cuts that total $150 billion per year? Eliminating these tax cuts would free up dollars to cover the uninsured and would help the federal deficit. In addition, just this year, the government "found" money for a number of "new important programs," like $94.5 billion for the wars in Iraq and Afghanistan, border security, hurricane relief, and pandemic flu preparedness. Again, it may be politically difficult to convince Congress or the American public to give up the tax breaks or to justify using any new federal dollars for health coverage expansions when there are other competing national needs like wars and natural disasters.

We know that the money to cover the uninsured, $83 billion and counting, is there on paper, in a variety of direct and indirect ways: government programs, private insurance cost shifting, and through tax subsidies. But is the money truly "available"? Not likely, given our current climate. We will see why in Chapter 19.

V

THE FUTURE

⑲

MYTH: ALL OTHER DEVELOPED COUNTRIES PROVIDE HEALTH CARE COVERAGE FOR EVERYONE; WE SHOULD BE NO DIFFERENT

But we *are* different. We do not have a Canadian health care system because we are not Canadian. The Canadian credo is "peace, order, and good government." Our American credo—life, liberty, and the pursuit of happiness—is about freedom and individualism, and certainly has nothing to do with "good government." So who are we? It is important to ask that question because who we are as Americans and, indeed, how America works, will ultimately determine the structure and principles that guide the development of our healt care system. In exploring who we are, and the effect on our health care system, we can best describe ourselves by ten principles:

TEN PRINCIPLES OF AMERICA

Rugged Individualism

The uniquely American "rags to riches" story is set in the national self-image of idealism, opportunity, and sacrifice, with origins in the "Wild West" and the Depression, in which one "pulled oneself up by the bootstraps" to get wealthy. The emphasis was on individual effort and responsibility in order to "make it." Such individualism extends to problem solving: "I don't need you to tell me what to do. I create my approach to solving problems, recognizing there may be a number of different ways to solve it. No reason we can't all do our own thing. I am a rugged individual."

"Rugged individualism" means different things to different people: in today's world, "making it" for a large number of people is not achieving wealth, but simply finding a paying job. Those who insist that "everyone can make it the way I did" might be surprised to know that about eighty percent of the uninsured live in families headed by workers, have to put bread on the table and a roof over their head, and the vast majority cannot afford health insurance despite working as hard as they can. But the myth lives on, "I'm not going to help you because you shouldn't need my help either."

Effect on the health care system. Since we think everyone should be able to "make it," we are reluctant to provide our tax dollars to support someone else's health care. We are charitable as individuals to individuals; we will help our neighbors and will take a sick, uninsured co-worker to the emergency room and might even pay for the visit. We perform amazing acts of kindness and humanitarian assistance in the face of natural disasters like Hurricane Katrina. But we have no interest in supporting large groups of "faceless" people, such as the uninsured, over the long term. The "I can do it myself" philosophy is the basis for today's emphasis on consumer-directed health care where individuals are "empowered" to make decisions for themselves, not taking into account how those decisions might affect the larger community. We like what we call "freedom of choice" to choose—and keep—our own doctors. We therefore are tolerant of multiple approaches to health care, which in turn permits (and reinforces) an extremely uncoordinated system.

Entrepreneurial

We will make money doing virtually anything; we value capitalism and the power of economic markets. We define success in monetary terms and as "the bottom line," whether an organization is called "for-profit" or "not-for-profit."

Effect on health care system. Like other industries, the business of health care values making money. We will continue to have insurance companies, as well as drug and device manufacturers, that are in the Fortune 500. Because profit is a measure of success, we will continue to have for-profit hospitals, for-profit doctors and for-profit lawyers, and not-for-profit organizations that look more and more like for-profit entities. Just like their for-profit counterparts, executives in the not-for-profit sector will be rewarded monetarily for their achievements. As a case in point, currently, CEOs at the six largest non-profit, tax-exempt hospital systems all make more than $1.2 million per year. We make a lot more money than our worldwide counterparts and it shows; it is the main reason our medical care is so expensive.

Simple Message Personalized to Me

The media is very powerful in "priming" us for certain messages or in the demand for certain products and focus on the individual consumer. Most marketing communications are written to make it seem like the message is "speaking to me directly," and the language is carefully chosen to give a short and simple "personalized message." Often, the fifteen-second "sound bite" is all that is needed to buy into the message, and this subtle (and sometimes not so subtle) manipulation connects us, personally, to whatever the message represents.

Effect on the health care system. When it comes to complex medical information, Americans want something simple. For example, the concept of "quality medical care" is extremely complicated, and so Americans prefer instead to use the "fix my car for the cheapest price" analogy when shopping for health insurance or medical care coverage. Rather than rely on expert information, we take the recommendation of our neighbor to choose our physician.

White Teeth

Remember, we live in a country founded on "the pursuit of happiness." This translates into, "I can have everything—white teeth (probably even white straight teeth), and a fancy automobile, and I can have it all now. I don't take no for an answer."

Effect on the health care system. We feel we have a "right" to whatever makes us happy and, therefore, we have a "right" to health care, all that we want. Americans feel entitled to any available medical service, regardless of its direct benefit. We will not wait for a physician visit and will become angry if we do not receive a return phone call within minutes. Waiting lines? Absurd. Rationing—no way.

Optimistic

"I can beat the odds. I will live through this." Americans and their loved ones are always the exception. Statistics are too complicated (see "Simple Message").

Effect on the health care system. A number of years ago a system was created that predicted with ninety-five-percent certainty whether an individual would leave an intensive care unit alive. It performed perfectly but was never accepted. Why? It failed because the patients' families were all convinced that their relative was in the five percent who would live. This is why we spend so much in the last twelve months of life. In many Americans' minds, death is not an option.

"It's the Economy, Stupid"

Our own personal finances as well as the economy of the country drives our views in so many areas. During the first presidential campaign of Bill Clinton, a sign hung in his campaign headquarters with the words, "It's the economy, stupid," to remind everyone working on the campaign that the American public goes into the voting booth thinking mainly about their own personal economic well-being.

Effect on the health care system. In a good economy with high employment, fewer people are uninsured (because more employers are able to offer insurance, and workers have more money to purchase it), and the issue of health insurance coverage disappears from the headlines. In a poor economy, levels of unemployment and uninsurance increase. As the economy continues to worsen, employers reduce the amount they are willing to pay for health insurance, either dropping coverage entirely or shifting more payment to the employee who is less able to pay the premiums. These actions increase the growing numbers of the uninsured.

The Thirty-to-Fifty-Year Liberal-Conservative Cycle

In recent times, the attitudes of Americans cycle every thirty to fifty years from liberal to conservative and back again. In a conservative world, private ownership is "king," taxes are low, government is small, individual freedom and responsibility reign, and there is a deep belief in "traditional values." Conversely, liberalism chooses the collective welfare of a society over the needs of the individual, and looks to government to protect the disadvantaged (usually through public programs paid for by taxing the "advantaged"), to curb capitalism, and to promote social justice.

Effect on the health care system. It is clear from history that overall social and economic conditions have a highly significant effect on how we feel about our health care system at any given time. This is also true with regard to our willingness to tolerate the number of people without insurance in this country and how much we challenge the status quo. Our current prevailing view of health care insurance favors continued involvement of the employer and supports only very slight incremental changes in our "system," if any at all, suggesting we are in a more conservative mode. However, there have been times in the past when America's views were more liberal, such as in the early 1960s when two sweeping social programs occurred: Medicare and Medicaid. The possibility for major change will occur about as often as the political merry-go-round passes the liberal brass ring.

Diversity

We are a country built on diversity and thriving on diversity. We have coffee bars on both coasts and right-to-life in the middle. In political terms, we have "red" and "blue" states. Since we are so different, it is no surprise that on average the country is average, and our elected officials must appeal to a wide variety of individuals who have varying interests and priorities. Given this marvelous diversity, agreeing on any large-scale national change is much less likely than incremental steps that offend the least number of people. Within each state, there is a bit more similarity among its citizens, bringing greater opportunities to advance more significant change that, at least, fits that particular state.

Effect on the health care system. With such diverse attitudes, many different types of systems are tolerated and even thrive, depending upon the political and economic environment. States that have a more homogeneous population (for example, Maine and Minnesota) are more likely to take on initiatives that advance a particular goal, such as reducing the number of the uninsured in their state. States are laboratories for change, and many experts believe that letting states experiment with programs that address health care coverage and cost problems within their boundaries will be more feasible than large-scale efforts for the entire country, at least in the short term.

Mistrust of Government

"I don't need federal or state bureaucrats who have their jobs for life (or those politicians who spend more of their time getting reelected than worrying about me) telling me what to do and spending my money. I certainly don't need to give them any more money—no more taxes." Sound familiar? Our ethic of "rugged individualism" applies here as an attitude that is anti-tax and anti-government.

Effect on our health care system. With this generalized mistrust of the federal government, employers as well as many individuals do not want government mandates to provide health care or to purchase health coverage for themselves. We do not want a "government-run" health care system. We point our fingers at Canada and their "government-run" program with "all those waiting lines and people coming to Detroit for medical care." Americans criticize Canada's centralized system, even as they praise our own Medicare program, which, in many ways, looks very similar to Canada's medical care system. We often read about seniors saying, "I don't want a government system—but don't take my Medicare away!" which doesn't make sense. But to most Americans, Medicare really isn't seen as a government program, even though the government pays the bills, because there is free choice of physician, free choice of where to go to the hospital, relatively short waiting times and now even prescription drugs. In fact, Medicare may not even be seen as a government-paid system, since it is really like Social Security, where "I paid for all those years into a Medicare account. I'm really using those dollars to pay for my health care."

A Unique Government

Lobbyists. Our government thrives on lobbyists; the vast majority of those who lobby the government do so for the same reasons: a desire for higher net income, lower taxes, and, for some, an improvement in quality of life—theirs. The most powerful lobbying groups in the United States are those representing medical care, technology, finance, and business groups like the Chambers of Commerce and the National Federation of Independent Businesses. In 2004, almost $2 billion was spent on federal lobbying, with the health care sector spending more than any other—$325 million. Many powerful groups of lobbyists, such as the pharmaceutical, medical device industry, and insurance companies, are directly involved in medical care, as are direct medical care providers, such as physicians and hospitals. While not directly a health care group, the American Association of Retired Persons (AARP) certainly has health care as one of its major agenda items and is very influential with Congress because of the large voting block represented by senior citizens.

Effect on health care system. These groups are likely to influence policy for long into the future because they provide generous campaign contributions for those running for office, or, like the AARP, they represent large blocks of voters. Those who ignore them lose.

Checks, balances, and partisanship. The way the Senate and House of Representatives are configured, consensus is required at many steps. Multiple committees with different rules (and certainly different members with different viewpoints) must all agree to a particular bill. Not only does each house have to agree, but so do the president and on occasion (usually much later) the Supreme Court. Given that each of these four bodies may—or may not be—of similar minds and similar parties, consensus may be easier or harder to reach. There is also a practical reason that elected officials favor incremental rather than comprehensive actions: most political candidates were elected on a platform of specific issues, and they run the risk of losing these supporters if things change too quickly or too much

Effect on the health care system. Incremental health care legislation is more likely than sweeping change, mainly because of the many different groups that make up and benefit from the existing system. As Machiavelli once noted, "It must be remembered that there is nothing more difficult to plan, more doubtful of success, nor more dangerous to manage, than the creation of a new system. For the initiator has the enmity of all who would profit by the preservation of the old institutions and merely lukewarm defenders in those who would gain by the new ones." Incremental change tries to bridge, slowly, the losses of the "old order" with the creation of new gains.

State vs. federal. In the United States, the levels of government are divided between the federal and state governments. There are strict rules about state and federal jurisdiction. States are required to balance their budgets, whereas the federal government is not, which means that states are more limited in the financial investments they can make. However, states are natural laboratories of change because they can at times circumvent the legislative gridlock at the federal government level and thus be more innovative and responsive to their individual state needs.

Effect on the health care system. The federal government has major power over taxation and the federal support programs of Medicare and Medicaid. There are key *federal* regulations that govern health care such as the Employee Retirement Income Security Act (ERISA) and the Health Insurance Portability and Accountability Act (HIPAA). ERISA frees large self-insured employers from state insurance regulations (which means most state health insurance regulation is for small businesses), and HIPAA eliminates pre-existing condition exclusions (but does not establish insurance rates) for workers in group health plans. On the other hand, states regulate the licensing of doctors and medical malpractice liability rules. States also determine many of the benefits within the Medicaid program, which has substantial variation from state to state because states often "add on" to the basic federal requirements—such as coverage of all aged people under one hundred percent of the Federal Poverty Level. Because states have different needs, state-based approaches to health care have been more popular, generally through securing waivers from the federal government to make changes in existing state programs, yet still relying on federal dollars for funding. There has been tremendous variation in state approaches and while some of these state-level changes have been popular, the requirement that states balance their budgets each year has caused long-term instability of new programs as the economic environment changes. In a good economy, there may be innovative state programs that support greater health coverage through a Medicaid program expansion or support of public-private initiatives that expand private insurance for workers in small business. Alternately, as the economy worsens, the states tighten their budgets, new programs are discontinued, and those who previously had health insurance may lose it.

CHARACTERISTICS OF THE AMERICAN HEALTH CARE SYSTEM BASED ON AMERICAN VALUES

Any health care system reform in the United States will have to reflect the underlying principles, values, and politics that make us who we are. This is not easy, partially because the interests are so varied and may be, at times, contradictory. Even so, at a minimum, any U.S. health care system will need to reflect the following:

1. Consistent with desires of the lobbyists;
2. Agreeable to private insurance companies;
3. Accommodate for-profit businesses and professions like drug and device industry, doctors, and lawyers;
4. Provide choice; and
5. I can have it all: little or no waiting for services; no rationing.

These first five are likely to be with us for quite some time. The next five may change, depending upon where we find ourselves in the liberal-conservative cycle:

6. No government mandates;
7. Continuation of employer-sponsored health care;
8. No centralized government-run system;
9. Not my tax dollars; and
10. At least a limited right to health care for everyone.

Not only will these American characteristics need to be satisfied in order to accomplish some kind of change in our health care system; but also the sun, moon, and the stars in the liberal-conservative cycle must also be aligned. Does that mean that change in the American health care system is impossible? We will explore this question in the next chapter.

20

MYTH: MAJOR CHANGE IN THE AMERICAN HEALTH CARE SYSTEM IS IMPOSSIBLE

There is a story about a man who knocks on the pearly gates, and St. Peter tells him he can ask one question. The man asks, "When will the United States have a rational health care system?" St. Peter stops and thinks and says, "Not in my lifetime!"

Well, we don't believe that. Why are people telling that story? It seems that all the way back to the beginning of the last century, individual presidents from both political parties have tried to change the entire health care system and have failed. The latest attempt was in 1993, the Health Security Act (HSA) proposed by the Clinton administration, and yet again America failed to support comprehensive "rational health care system" reform.

PREVIOUS PLANS FAILED BECAUSE THEY FORGOT WHO WE ARE

Why did this latest attempt fail? If we go back to Chapter 19 and look at the ten characteristics of American health care based on American values and how they might be applied to a national health reform plan, the failure of the HSA can be better understood.

Consistent with the desires of the lobbyists. First of all, influential special interest groups were not included in the initial planning. The task force consisted of outsiders and left out the most "influential special interest group" in the country: the U.S. Congress, as well as other Washington, D.C., "insiders." Clearly, they also largely left out other powerful "interest" groups such as the pharmaceutical industry, the insurance industry, and physicians.

Agreeable to private insurance companies. The role of independent insurance companies was minimized under the plan, and the health insurance industry attacked, leading one of the more successful advertising campaigns with the "Harry and Louise" commercials. These ads, geared toward the "average American," showed a husband and wife with worried looks and voices discussing how a government-run health care system would take away their current level of health care.

Accommodate for-profit businesses and professionals like drug and device industry, doctors, and lawyers. The Health Security Act also included a national budget for health care set by the Congress, which meant there would be a fixed amount of money set aside each year for health care spending. Having a fixed budget for total health expenditures created fear on the part of various health industries; fear that research into innovative drugs would be squashed as too expensive or that payments to physicians and hospitals would be reduced year after year to meet the budget. Even the lawyers lost.

Provide choice. The reform plan favored health maintenance organizations (HMOs) with limited choice of physician, something that was very unpopular with most Americans. In health care, being able to choose one's own physician and easy referral to a specialist are very important. Limiting choice, to many in the United States, is considered to be taking something away that is theirs.

I can have it all: little or no waiting for services; no rationing. Patients became concerned that the plan would result in waiting lists so common in England and Canada. Americans did not want to wait months for hip replacement, heart surgery, or even a visit to the doctor. With the plan's limited budget, the fear of rationing became closer to reality. Public opinion polls consistently demonstrated that Americans wanted more medical care, not less, and this still holds true today.

No government mandates. Under the Health Security Act, individuals were required to have health care coverage and all businesses were required to contribute. These requirements were viewed as unpopular government "mandates" and invited plenty of opposition from individuals and businesses who felt they could not afford health insurance. This may not always be a problem (depending upon the conservative-liberal cycle) as we have recently seen in Massachusetts, but it was a problem then.

Continuation of employer-sponsored health insurance. Employers sponsor the vast majority of health insurance. It has become traditional for businesses to use this benefit as a recruitment tool and to "buy" the long-term loyalty of employees. Under the Health Security Act, only the largest employers were permitted to insure their own employees, leaving the rest, and the majority, of employers cut off from these advantages.

No centralized government-run system. The proposed system was highly regulated by the government. The term "managed competition" was used under the Health Security Act, presumably so it would not sound quite so government-controlled and appeal to free market proponents. Even so, the plan's "managed competition" insurance model was viewed as putting government controls in place to "manage" the market-based competition among private health plans and was ultimately rejected as "government-run."

Not with my tax dollars. The financing of the new system was difficult to explain, and because it was more expensive, at least in the short term, it was easier for the American public to oppose the need for new taxes than to focus on any potential long-term savings that might have resulted from a more efficient system.

At least a limited right to health care for everyone. At the beginning of the debate in 1990, the fact that there were thirty-seven million uninsured shocked everyone into action; by the end in 1993, the fact that there were "only" thirteen percent of the population (and that eighty-six percent had insurance) was taken as reassuring. The fact that thirty-seven million *is* thirteen percent, and that those were the same number, escaped people, but they used a different rationale at the end to say that we don't really have to have health care for everyone—we're doing pretty well.

The complexity, cost, and comprehensiveness of the Health Security Act gave everyone in the Congress something to hate. The proposed legislation certainly was not simple. Diagrams were produced pointing out the similarity of the plan to the complexity of the New York subway system and it was difficult to personalize the plan for the individual voter. During the debate, less than twenty percent of Americans said that they even had a basic understanding of what was being proposed.

Major reform is difficult to get through the Congressional committee process in the best of times. All it takes is a few well-placed individuals to derail the process, and, ultimately, that was the fate of the Clinton administration's attempt to reform the U.S. health system. Despite a popular president and a congress of the same party, an opportunity for comprehensive health care reform did not occur in 1994, just as it did not in 1948, 1965, and 1974, and for many of the same reasons. There are political lessons here. Interestingly, as we shall see, despite the failure of the Health Security Act, many of its principles were sound and we have seen some used in recent state legislation.

BAD AND GETTING WORSE

But despite failed attempts, we must do something. Over five million working Americans have lost health coverage since 2000 and one in four poor Americans under the age of sixty-five report being uninsured for at least four years. Between now and 2013, personal spending on health care is estimated to increase 7.4 percent per year while personal income will increase 4.6 percent per year. Every one-percent increase in personal health care spending above the rate of growth in personal income increases the number of uninsured each year by 246,000. At this rate, there will be at least fifty-six million uninsured Americans by 2013, representing almost twenty percent of the U.S. population.

In 2004, eighty-seven percent of Americans said that legislation to provide health insurance to the uninsured was "extremely important." In fact, most of us agree on the overall concepts and goals that will move us toward a reformed health care system.

CONCEPTS AND GOALS FOR REFORM

Most Americans agree on some variation of the following concepts and goals.

Health coverage for all Americans. Along with the forty-six million Americans without health insurance, another sixteen million are "underinsured," which means that their health insurance does not protect them adequately because their medical expenses exceed ten percent of income. Over the course of one year, thirty-five percent of people nineteen to sixty-four years old in this country had either no insurance or were underinsured.

High quality, necessary medical care with shared responsibility. We have defined "high quality" medical care in Chapter 9: safe, effective, efficient, timely, patient-centered, and equitable. High quality care involves a partnership between the physician and the patient where each shares responsibility for treatment decisions. Patients must take responsibility for their own unhealthy behaviors and physicians must view care from the patient's perspective and be able to give patients important information in understandable language.

Controlling health care costs. Clearly, elimination of waste is paramount in defining a reformed system, and to this end, competition with rewards for efficient, high-value care is important. Defining "medically necessary" care is not always easy because we currently give too little care to some people and too much care to others. Looking to data on what the best practices are, what works, and what is truly "necessary" will be key in a reformed system.

Administrative simplification. The amount of money it takes to "run" our hybrid private/public health system accounts for nearly thirty percent of national health expenditures. Health care "administrative expenses" include items such as billing, advertising, compliance with regulations, management of employer plans, the administrative costs of health care providers, and the plan's "profit." These different functions across so many different private and public insurance providers promote excess paperwork and create a fragmented and inefficient "system." Today, nearly forty percent of the eighteen billion transactions that occur in the health care system still happen on paper. Reducing billing costs and other administrative efficiencies could save $60 billion a year.

Public-private solutions with adequate financial assistance. Any solutions that move us toward a new framework on which to build our health care system will need to involve private and public systems as well as financial support to make it affordable for individuals, business, and the nation.

AN APPROACH TO CHANGE

We have made suggestions on how to improve quality and cost in previous chapters, and we now will concentrate on how to improve coverage. It is

important to note, however, that improving coverage cannot occur in isolation. We must improve quality, cost, and coverage all together because their
success is linked: in improving costs, we must not allow quality to suffer; by
curbing the growth of cost, we will be able to afford better coverage for the
uninsured.

Let's review the current ways in which Americans obtain health care coverage; the simplest way to approach this is to think of five major "pieces" of
a puzzle. These are provided in greater detail in chapters 14 and 16:

Medicare. This federal program covers those over sixty-five years of age,
as well as others such as the disabled. The system of care is efficient (three
percent administrative costs) and has widespread patient satisfaction. In
fact, Medicare enrollees are more satisfied, generally, than younger Americans in private plans.

The Veterans Administration (VA) Medical Center. The VA, which
provides care to those who have served in the armed forces, is the country's
largest integrated delivery system and is leading the nation in innovative
programs aimed at the reduction of medical errors and introduction of electronic medical records.

Employer-based insurance for very large employers. Very large
employers—those with 1,000 employees or more—are almost always self-
insured, have great knowledge of the health care system, and are able to influence change through their purchasing power. Typically, these large employers have a health insurance benefits infrastructure that provides
economies of scale with multiple choices of plans. These programs are very
popular with workers. Employees in large companies also change jobs less frequently, making loss of health care continuity by changing jobs less likely.

Employer-based insurance for smaller employers. The percentage of
small employers offering health benefits has been falling since 2000, largely
because of the expense of offering health insurance. Health insurance costs
eighteen percent more in small businesses for the same level of coverage, and
often employees pay a greater share of the premium. Among those with less
than 200 employees, only fifty-nine percent of employees are offered health
insurance. In general, low-wage workers employed in small firms are least
likely to have employee benefits and are most likely to be uninsured. Less
than half of those who make under $20,000 per year have health insurance.

The "safety net" programs. Medicaid, the State Children's Health Insurance Program (SCHIP), and support for Federally Qualified Health

Centers are the largest combined federal and state programs that pay for health care to the uninsured and to the rural poor. They complement the care provided by Academic Health Centers, state hospitals, and county hospitals that give care to residents within a particular state or county. In combination, all of these programs have been described by optimists as a "patchwork" of services and, alternately, by pessimists as an "uncoordinated sieve" that allows many of the forty-six million uninsured to fall through the "safety net."

Based on these different ways in which Americans receive health care coverage, what approaches might be possible to increase health coverage? For the time being, let us assume that the lessons of history are true: that incremental changes to improve the system are more politically feasible than comprehensive change. If this is the case, then leaving three of the five health coverage areas relatively unchanged would be prudent. Medicare, the Veterans' Administration system, and employer-based insurance for very large employers all seem to be working pretty well for those who are in them. The funding of these systems is going to be increasingly inadequate over time, but as systems of care, they work relatively well. Conversely, the other two areas, employer-based insurance for smaller employers and safety net programs, are not working especially well for those obtaining health coverage through them. Therefore, it makes sense to consider ways they could change.

ATTEMPTS TO IMPROVE OPTIONS FOR SMALL BUSINESS

If every person who worked in a small business (and their families) had health insurance, the uninsured would decrease by sixty percent. There are two factors standing in the way: (1) inefficiency of providing health care through small business, and (2) funding. There have been numerous recent attempts in different states to address both inefficiency and affordability to improve insurance coverage for employees in small businesses. It has become absolutely clear that both approaches are needed simultaneously.

Inefficiencies. First we need to address the inefficiencies in providing health insurance to small businesses. It is clear that marketing to and serving large numbers of businesses with small numbers of employees are inefficient. The first strategy to deal with inefficiency would allow a "pooling"

mechanism in which small employers could join together in order to negotiate health insurance prices as a larger unit. One such pooling program,
Healthy New York, was developed as a public/private insurance program
that offers health insurance benefits to small companies, the self-employed,
and workers who cannot obtain insurance from an employer. The state
funds a "stop loss" part of the program; in other words, the state covers all
medical costs for an individual above a certain amount. Healthy NY is a
state-subsidized reinsurance program that reimburses health plans for
ninety percent of the claims paid between $5,000 and $75,000 in a calendar
year. This, in turn, permits the health insurance premiums to remain affordable. Established in 2001, enrollment in 2005 reached 100,000. Fifty-
seven percent of enrollees are working individuals, and twenty-five percent
are enrolled through small employer groups. Most members subscribing to
Healthy NY pay thirty to fifty percent less for their premiums than for similar coverage in the individual market and fifteen to thirteen percent less
than rates in the small group market. For example, monthly Healthy NY
HMO individual premiums averaged around $200 dollars per month com-
pared with $340 for private individual market premiums.

Although the idea of pooling small businesses in order to share risk and
assume market power seems like an attractive option, pools have their problems as well. One study suggests that insurance pools do not in fact lower
premiums nor decrease the number of uninsured workers despite the appeal and logic of pooling. There are two main reasons put forward why
pools may not work: 1) Small employers and the self-employed have the
choice to leave a pool if the cost of health coverage becomes too expensive.
Therefore, pools may suffer from "adverse selection" because the small
businesses that choose to remain in the pools may have sicker employees
who need health coverage. 2) Unless a pool can attract and maintain a large
number of people, it will not achieve economies of scale nor be able to negotiate with health plans.

The second strategy is to allow individuals (rather than small businesses)
to pool risk by allowing them to join larger insurance pools such as a Federal Employees' Health Benefits Program (FEHBP). In the current FE-
HBP program, individual governmental employees receive once per year,
in the mail or on the web, information describing the health plans available
in the geographic area in which they live and work. A report card that describes each health plan is made available to each employee, with compar-

ative ratings that measure everything from patient satisfaction to clinical outcomes, such as coronary artery bypass mortality (see Chapter 9). The employee decides which plan he or she wants to participate in (either for themselves or for themselves and their family), and the employer (in this case the federal government) pays its share every month while the required amount from the employee is automatically deducted from their paycheck. This is the same system used in most state employee health plans as well, with large numbers of employees pooled in order to spread the risk. If individuals and small businesses were allowed to buy into the large governmental employee pool (either federal or state), they could choose from among the available plans offered through the governmental program and take advantage of the lower premiums and more stable coverage than those available to individuals and small businesses.

Affordability. Despite efforts at pooling, affordability for small business continues to be a major issue. Lack of funding has been the major reason given for the low enrollment in many pools to date.

Even if pools were able to get the price of insurance as low as the price for large businesses, premiums must be paid by a combination of the employer and the employee to make it affordable for workers. Studies have suggested that a thirty-percent subsidy to the employee will only yield a three-percent increase in the number of small business employees with insurance. In most models, the subsidy to the employee needs to be sixty to sixty-seven percent by either the employee or the government or both.

Low wage earners on average are willing to pay one or two percent of their income for health coverage, approximately $900 per year for a low-income family of four. It is likely that small business owners would also match that for a total of $1,800 per year. For a "bare bones" plan, approximately $3,000 would be required for an individual and $6,000 for a family, therefore leaving a required subsidy of $1,200 for an individual and $4,200 for a family. In this case, a subsidy would be required from the government. Nationally, the Bush administration has proposed a tax credit of $1,000 for an individual and $3,000 for a family, but this is not likely to be enough to make health insurance affordable for low-income workers. However, the point here is that a policy has been developed to support a mechanism for this kind of subsidy and therefore should be pursued as a policy option to expand coverage for low-income workers.

Such subsidies have now been tried at the state level as well. In two different models in Michigan, a "three-share" approach—in which employers, workers, and the government each pay about one-third of the cost of health care—has been used to expand health coverage to low-income workers in small businesses. In one program, Health Choice, low-income small businesses with more than three workers are eligible to participate in the program so long as employers live and work in the county. Workers who make $10 an hour or less are eligible for the full one-third government-share subsidy, while workers who make more receive less. In addition, as recently as June 2006, the governor of Tennessee signed legislation entitled Cover Tennessee, providing a state-subsidized health plan for hard-to-insure adults and some of the more than 600,000 Tennessean workers and their families who are uninsured. Like the Michigan program, Cover Tennessee spreads the cost of health insurance among the employee, the employer, and the state, and current estimates are that 100,000 adults, 75,000 children, and 15,000 chronically ill low-income individuals will enroll over the next three years.

State as the "backup." State "high-risk pools" have been tried by states as a means of providing health insurance to those whose health conditions make it difficult for them to obtain health coverage. They have been around for twenty-five years, and in 2004 covered 172,000 people in thirty-four states. However, despite their potential to provide a safety net for sicker-than-average individuals, the high premiums, deductibles, and co-payments severely limit the impact of high-risk pools in making insurance available and affordable. Even with state subsidies (and most states do not offer financial assistance), premiums average around $5,000 for an individual, making it unaffordable for the vast majority. In fact, in most states, only one to two percent of the eligible population is covered by these high risk pools. The idea of the state becoming a "back-up" by capping the liability of a plan through reinsurance has been tried in New York, as mentioned above. The concept of reinsurance has recently re-emerged as a potential mechanism to support small-group and individual health coverage. When states assume a portion of insurers' high-cost claims, premiums are lower, more stable, and the benefits more generous. Several states have explored the use of state-subsidized reinsurance programs, similar to the New York program, to improve access to health insurance.

Reduce price or benefits. Other public policies have been proposed that would reduce the price of benefits or reduce the actual benefits provided to make health insurance affordable for small businesses. Many states have insurance laws that require health plans to offer certain benefits, which can drive up the cost of the premiums. Federal legislation has been introduced to promote the formation of Association Health Plans (AHPs), where small businesses would band together to offer health insurance without having to comply with state insurance benefit regulations. The goal of AHPs is to lower the cost of insurance by permitting reduced benefits. But critics of AHPs point out that consumer protections like emergency room coverage or specialized services for diabetics will not be covered in AHPs: stripped-down, "bare bones" insurance policies are appealing to small businesses with low-wage employees because they are less costly, but often they sacrifice access to needed health care services. AHPs may also promote adverse selection: companies with the healthiest workers could migrate to the lower-cost, lower-benefit Association Health Plans, leaving the sickest in traditional, state-regulated insurance plans, which now would be forced to raise premiums without the healthier workers in the risk pool.

The other currently popular way of decreasing the price of benefits is the high-deductible plan, in which the employee pays the first $1,000 to $2,000 (or more) of expenses. While attractive in terms of price, there may be problems: (1) the individual is unable to pay the deductible, and therefore providers are not paid; (2) the individual may "hoard" the deductible for a rainy day so that the appropriate preventive care, or even follow-up care for chronic disease, is not sought. High out-of-pocket costs are a particularly difficult problem for lower-income families; twenty-nine percent of adults with incomes below $20,000 spend more than five percent of their income on out-of-pocket health care costs. As discussed in Chapter 10, if high-deductible health plans are viewed as a possible option for employees in small businesses, easily accessed good information along with consumer education will be necessary to help individuals spend their money wisely and shop wisely for health plans.

ATTEMPTS TO IMPROVE THE SAFETY NET

We will always need a safety net. Most attempts to improve the safety net in recent years have been individual states expanding Medicaid and/or the State Children's Health Insurance Program (SCHIP). The first "expansions" increased enrollment for people who are already eligible for these programs. For example, approximately twenty-five percent of children who are eligible for Medicaid and SCHIP are not enrolled. This can be changed with aggressive state actions. Since all kids under 200 percent of the Federal Poverty Level are eligible for coverage under either SCHIP or Medicaid, the goal should be that no low-income child should be without health coverage instead of the (2002) uninsurance rate of seventeen percent for low-income kids. Thirty-seven percent of low-income adults are uninsured and some states have been pursuing Medicaid and SCHIP expansions, copying Tennessee's Medicaid expansion, TennCare, to cover adults under 100 percent of poverty. Unfortunately, while the concept was sound, administrative problems caused tremendous problems for TennCare. A number of states expanded their covered populations either through Medicaid or SCHIP, only to reduce them when state budgets could not support the coverage expansions.

A different approach to cover uninsured adults is to expand Medicare to early retirees or to those between the ages of fifty-five and sixty-four. There is evidence that extending insurance coverage to this population would improve health and survival, and reduce their health care spending during that nine-year period. It has the ability to improve health and to spread risk among an existing large pool of enrollees, and coupled with Medicare's low administrative costs, may be a viable recommendation for the hard-to-insure fifty-five to sixty-four year olds who are without health coverage. Bringing in adults earlier to the Medicare program would actually be an expansion of the "single-payer" methodology, because Medicare is a single-payer system for the elderly in this country.

WHERE DO WE GO FROM HERE?

Near-Term: Incremental Change

Changes in coverage: Start with the states. While the American public wants something done—they routinely rank health care as one of the top three issues for government to address—they are equally divided on which approach to choose: expanding private insurance through small business with subsidies, expanding public programs that help the low-income like Medicaid and SCHIP, or expanding a single payer like Medicare.

Instead of choosing one, we should consider providing incremental improvement in all three areas: (1) methodology for pooling of small business and access to pools for individuals such as the Federal Employee Health Benefit Program or State Employees plans, with state reinsurance, and subsidies above a certain income level so that no one pays more than 2.5–7.5 percent of income for health care; (2) expansion of Medicaid and SCHIP, perhaps to those under 200 to 300 percent of the Federal Poverty Level; and (3) Medicare expansion to cover those fifty-five years of age and above.

We should start with the states. Since we are currently in an "incremental mode" and are not likely, at least in the next several years, to enact sweeping methodology for overall expansion, it seems reasonable to propose innovation in all three of these methods (or others) at the level of the states. The Institute of Medicine as well as Harvard researchers have recommended this approach. Federal legislation has recently been introduced to support state innovation: the Health Partnership Act would provide federal grants to states that propose innovative ways to improve coverage, quality and efficiency. States have demonstrated that they are outstanding proving grounds. For example, Massachusetts has recently passed legislation by an overwhelming majority that involves health insurance mandates that require all individuals to have health insurance and requires all businesses to contribute—something from the Clinton Health Security Act that we thought unlikely to work a decade ago. As it becomes apparent which approaches are the most effective, other states, and eventually the country, can learn.

Changes in cost: it's the money, stupid. All the structure in the world will not work if we don't address the cost of medical care. We are left with the problem that will not go away: there is more medical care out there than we can afford, and the availability and expense will get worse. Some say that this really isn't a problem: We are a wealthy country, and can easily spend even twenty percent or twenty-five percent of GDP on medical care. Such spending would be expected as we age and the economy grows. At our current spending levels, we are projected to reach twenty percent of GDP by 2015. Remember, in addition to other cost-drivers, if we are successful in covering the uninsured, it will cost an additional $83 billion. The problem with this thinking is that every dollar spent on health is a dollar not available to spend on other national programs that are also important to us, programs such as education, defense, Social Security, or energy. What can we do?

How much money is in the system? The "areas of potential opportunity" identified in Chapter 18 include elimination of the tax deduction given to employers for health care, or a rollback of the current tax cuts. When individuals are asked which areas are "very important" to fund if there were ever a rollback, seventy-four percent say health care, but seventy-three percent say education, fifty-nine percent Social Security, and fifty-nine percent the environment. In 2003, forty-three percent of Americans said we should "increase taxes substantially if it is the only way to be sure that every American got needed health care." About $250 per taxpayer (individual or family) would be required to achieve the $83 billion. Remember in Chapter 18 we discussed how Americans are already "paying" for much of the uninsured's care in higher health insurance premiums. The $250 per taxpayer is already in the system. If we can't squeeze it out initially, then perhaps it would be possible to pass the costs of insuring workers on to business as their productivity increases due to better health in their newly insured workers. Or perhaps we could pass it on to insurance companies as more workers would be in their plans and as their administrative costs decrease with electronic medical records and electronic billing. Of course, taxes could be raised with increases in "sin taxes" such as cigarettes, or even with a proposed "fatty food tax," where it has been estimated that a tax similar to that for cigarettes on foods with three grams or more of saturated fat would yield $83 billion for the country.

Eliminate waste. We spent all of Chapter 3 discussing how to reduce waste by both physicians and patients. We can improve our administrative systems and practice safer, more effective medicine, educating and re-educating physicians so that malpractice is markedly reduced, and work with patients to promote healthier lifestyles and adherence to medical recommendations, but these improvements alone will not solve the problem of continual cost increases. Improvements in information systems and administrative simplification will provide some efficiencies, but not enough, especially over time. All of the parts of medical spending are growing at a faster rate than the GDP, and they will continue to grow even if we were able to make cost reductions in any given year. Medical costs are driven by the price as well as the increased volume and intensity of services provided to patients, which together has consistently been higher than general inflation by about three percent each year for the last forty years. As in the past, future growth in medical spending will be linked to new technologies, more technologies per patient, increasing expectations of patients as the Baby Boom population ages, and the discovery and treatment of new diseases. In short, there are not enough administrative efficiencies or ways to eliminate waste in the system to balance the increase in volume and intensity of services or the increasing price of medical services. In addition, we had better get to work on increasing the medical care workforce; the reduced supply of physicians and nurses will cause labor prices to skyrocket, making the problem worse. Ultimately, we will have to make the hard choices about what we do without to control costs and preserve quality.

Tough decisions. We believe that we must begin to make tough decisions. It may surprise you to know that the government does not take into consideration what a treatment costs when deciding what is covered through the Medicare and Medicaid programs. As we said in Chapter 7, this must change: explicit decisions on what should be done must be based on how well it works (how much will each life improve, and how many lives will be improved) *and* what it costs. We can begin now by setting high bars for new drugs and devices: they should meet hurdles for really improving our lives, and we should compare the cost with current practice. Other developed countries already do this. As we get more used to the idea of analysis including cost, we should then look to our system and begin to make the very tough choices for how to do the best for the most in a world of economic reality. We are also mindful that every time a "tough decision" is reached, somebody is going to think that they lose—whether it is reducing the amount paid or reducing the amount done—and they will oppose change. In the near term, these tough decisions will be reached differently by different payers, but we must begin to reach them. We cannot all have it all.

INTERMEDIATE-TERM—2012–2019: A NATIONAL APPROACH

The state pilots should coalesce into a national approach with coverage for all. The characteristics of this approach will borrow from what will be shown to have worked in certain states. It will likely not be a single payer, but will have a floor of Medicaid/SCHIP, perhaps for all people up to three hundred percent of the Federal Poverty Level. Those above the three-hundred-percent Federal Poverty Level limit would buy private insurance either as individuals or as businesses, using pooling mechanisms similar to the

Federal Employee Health Benefits Program. The amount of the individual premium for basic benefits would need to be related to income, such that the premium did not exceed 2.5–7.5 percent of income. Since the premium would be affordable at this level, individuals would be required to purchase health insurance. The remainder of the premium would be contributed by either business (where the business would either be required to provide a certain level of insurance or pay a certain amount—so-called "pay-or-play") or government, perhaps with a tax credit.

THE LONG TERM—2020 AND BEYOND: SYSTEM CHANGE

Major restructuring must occur in the safety net. Ideally, there should be a single safety net including Medicare, Medicaid, and state and community programs. This should provide subsidized coverage for those up to a reasonable level of income where health care does not cost more than 2.5–7.5 percent of income. For those who are over fifty-five, a reduced premium for the safety net program would be available, although in some way also related to income. The system would have evidence-based benefits based on cost, effectiveness, and high quality care that reward physicians and hospitals who meet certain quality benchmarks. Because of the number of powerful interests in the health care sector (e.g., hospitals, physician groups, the insurance and pharmaceutical industries that are all prone to influence government), the establishment of an independent board would be necessary to make the tough decisions on what health services to include in the safety net coverage. Since an individual's contribution will be relatively fixed (related to income), and explicit subsidies will be required to cover the remainder of the cost, the coverage choices will have to be balanced within a defined budget. The amount this budget increases each year will be a matter for public debate.

The remainder of Americans could have a completely private system with its own insurance products. In the private system, the individual would have a broader range of private physicians, and "elective procedures" such as plastic surgery would be covered, but the goal would be that there would be similar health outcomes in the private system and the "basic" safety net system. In keeping with the American requirement for individual choice and preference, those in the private system could buy extra care that the basic system did not cover, such as very expensive drugs. This type of model would keep safe the American value of "buying up" and dispel the fear that it is socialized "government-run" health care.

WHAT WILL BE NECESSARY FOR THE SUN, MOON, AND STARS TO ALIGN?

What would need to occur to bring about our ideas for a rational health care system? Lobbyists and voters must demand it before politicians will enact it. How will that happen, and when?

Whatever "finger in the dike" strategy is in vogue at the time to reduce costs will run its course and be proven not to work in the long run. For example, the 1990s solution to the cost problem—HMOs—did not save money after several years. Similarly, we can imagine that today's "consumer-driven health plans" with Health Savings Accounts and high deductibles will be shown not to save money (and worse, will be shown to reduce access and quality as well).

Employer costs will increase or profits will decrease, despite shifting more health insurance premiums and medical care costs to employees. There will come a time when employers are ready to unload employer-sponsored insurance to protect their profit margin and their global competitive edge. The signal will be when the first large employer stops providing health benefits, or goes bankrupt, or both.

Proposals for a new system will occur at the time of an economic downturn, when we know that the number of Americans who will be unemployed and uninsured will rise. Different than the traditional uninsured who don't vote, a large segment of the newly uninsured will begin to target their votes. As more and more educated higher-income workers find health coverage unaffordable, they may be able to provide political pressure. This will occur sooner if the Baby Boomers sense that they are not getting the highest quality health care, and they will vote.

Over time, as the new generations of Americans, the "Gen X," and "Gen Y," begin to think more about themselves and their families, it is possible that with more time at home, they will begin to "talk over the back fence" with their neighbors and develop more of a sense of community.

Finally, maybe the health care reform merry-go-round will simply get to the right place in history, and social policy may move politics: we may decide that providing health care for all (and helping to pay for it) is the right thing to do, and a majority of us will vote for it. If the time is right and the interests align, voters will respond, likely around a presidential campaign. Stay tuned: when the voters, the lobbyists, the president, and the congress are aligned (and they will be), we will have a rational health care system.

> We should not accept without challenge what we know to be abominable just because it appears to be inevitable.
>
> —Jordan Cohen

AFTERWORD

When *Health Care Half-Truths: Too Many Myths, Not Enough Reality* was delivered to the publishers, national health care reform was just a long-forgotten dream, or nightmare, depending on one's perspective. Fast-forward six months and the 2008 presidential candidates of both parties were designing campaign platforms and delivering speeches about the problems in our health care system and the importance of national action. While we might have guessed this would be the case, it would have been difficult to anticipate the groundswell of attention over the last year regarding the need for national reform. For that reason, when writing *Health Care Half-Truths*, we ended the book knowing that a national program was absolutely necessary but would have to be developed over time, likely with input from state innovation.

For now, the states will continue to provide the leadership for health care reform efforts, much as we have seen in Massachusetts. The Massachusetts plan was as yet untested when we took *Health Care Half-Truths* to press, but we now have the "early returns" of what has worked in that plan, and, equally importantly, what has not worked. There are no real surprises: it is more expensive than they thought, and people are having a tough time paying for the mandated heath insurance. So much so, in fact,

60,000 Massachusetts residents of middle income have been given a waiver from the mandate.

Recently, some have said that it is "disloyal" to discuss state reform when national reform is on the agenda, but we disagree. State reforms will continue to be an "end" as well as a "means": the end will be insuring more Americans in the short-term and the means will be the creation of ideas and lessons we can carry into crafting a national solution. This will take time, and unfortunately there are no "cookie-cutter" remedies. In our view, any acceptable redesign of the national health care system will require the majority of Americans to weigh in for coverage for other people—and we are not there yet.

We predict that the myths we've introduced readers to in this book will be amplified in the coming months and year, not only as overly simplistic media sound bites that advance one reform over another, but also because Americans are less satisfied with the status quo and are increasingly demanding action. The challenge is to nudge Americans away from unrealistic and impossible solutions, as attractive as they may sound, and toward a better understanding of what will be required to enact a more rational health care system.

Despite all the current pronouncements (and our own hope for a national solution), we still believe comprehensive health care reform is a long shot in the short-term. No matter what happens after the next president is elected, the funding for significant reform is simply not there. We are still spending hundreds of billions of dollars overseas, and any savings that might be achieved through reducing administrative waste and by practicing medicine more efficiently are likely five years away before there is any new coverage for the uninsured. In the interim, signs point only to continued incremental measures: powerful interest groups will continue to advocate for the status quo, and among reformers, genuine philosophical differences will continue to be debated as to the value of public versus private solutions. Real change will not be easy, and, as we say at the end of the book, true reform will only come when the American people are ready and only when a president and Congress put this issue at the very top of the national agenda.

Articulating these reform options and making them understandable, or even agreeing that reform is necessary, is easy enough to state in the abstract but exceedingly difficult to achieve in the real world. Nevertheless, one thing is clear: each of us, in our own way, will have to work to bring real and lasting change to our dysfunctional health care system. *Health Care Half-Truths* promises to help readers sift through the facts and fiction surrounding the organization, financing, and delivery of health care in this country—the kind of information needed before tackling the broader issues of reform. Understanding the myths and realities in today's world of medicine and health care will lead to a greater national consciousness about what we can realistically expect from a health care system that must balance our needs and wants with what we can afford. Only then can we begin to shape a uniquely American system of health care that we are capable of achieving and that we all deserve.

Arthur Garson Jr. and Carolyn L. Engelhard
June 2008

SOURCES FOR THE FACTS
AND FURTHER READING

CHAPTER I

Health Care

Life Expectancy

U.S. Department of Health and Human Services, Centers for Disease Control and Prevention. National Vital Statistics System, National Vital Statistics Reports. Volume 53, Number 5: Deaths: Final Data for 2002, published October 14, 2004. This article presents information about trends and differences in death rates, infant mortality, and life expectancy by race. The article also compares trends relating to the leading causes of death for adults and infants, and the effects of socioeconomic characteristics.

National Center for Health Statistics. Health, United States, 2004. Washington DC: Government Printing Office. See also see National Center for Health Statistics website, http://www.cdc.gov/nchs/, for national mortality statistics and health trends in the U.S.

U.S. Department of Health and Human Services, Healthy People 2010, 2nd ed. Washington: U.S. Government Printing Office, November 2000. For chapters on Understanding and Improving Health, Objectives for Improving Health, and Systematic Approaches to Health Improvement, see

http://www.healthypeople.gov/Document/tableofcontents
.htm#uih. Healthy People 2010 is an initiative aimed at increasing life expectancy and quality of life, and eliminating health disparities for individuals and communities. This website has more information about the Healthy
People 2010 initiative and includes information about current life expectancy, infant mortality, and the relationships among health status and income, income and education, and ethnicity and education.

What Affects Health?

*Isaacs, S.L. and Schroeder, S.A. (2004). Class—The Ignored Determinant of
the Nation's Health. New England Journal of Medicine 351(11): 1137–1142.*
The authors discuss the relationship of health (in terms of life expectancy and
likelihood of disease) to social class and income distribution. Health determinants are made up of many social, economic, and biological factors, but health
reform efforts in the United States have focused primarily on the access to and
payment of medical insurance. Medical care has been estimated to delay premature death by only ten to fifteen percent, thus having little impact on the
overall health of a nation. The authors believe that in order to eliminate health
disparities, which will lead to greater improvements in health, we need to increase our understanding of the relationship between health and social class,
and develop social and economic policies to address the problem.

*Marmot, M. The Influence of Income on Health: Views of an Epidemiol-
ogist. Health Affairs 21(2) (March/April 2002): 31–46* discusses how income
is related to health. The author defines what is meant by a "social gradient"
in health, and discusses how personal income determines the extent to
which one can purchase health care, live in an environment that promotes
good health, and have control over one's life. The author also discusses past
studies to support his theory that income disparities within a society and between societies create poor health.

*Marmot, M. "Status Syndrome: A Challenge to Medicine." JAMA 295(11)
(2006): 1304–1307.* There is a social gradient in health: not only do the poor
have poor health, but even those who are not truly poor but who have lower
social position have poorer health. The higher the social position, the better the health. The author calls this the "status syndrome" in health, and reports that those with lower social status have increased risk of disease and
mortality. The stress that comes from a lack of control or autonomy in one's
occupation predisposes one to heart disease, absenteeism, and mental ill-

ness problems. The author concludes by saying that the "status syndrome" in American health care is an urgent social and medical problem.

Lurie, N. What the Federal Government Can Do About the Nonmedical Determinants of Health, Health Affairs 21(2) (March/April 2002): 94–105. The article discusses (and provides recommendations to the federal government) how the differences in income and education affect obesity and substance abuse.

Henry J. Kaiser Family Foundation (2005). Policy Challenges and Opportunities in Closing the Racial Ethnic Divide in Health Care, Publication No. 7293. This issue brief discusses the evidence for racial/ethnic differences in medical care and ways to close the gap and promote quality health care. See many resources on health disparities at the Kaiser Family Foundation website: www.kff.org.

Institute of Medicine, Unequal Treatment: Confronting Racial and Ethnic Disparities in Health Care, Washington: National Academy Press, 2002. This study by the Institute of Medicine looks at the issue of racial and ethnic disparities in health care, in terms of access factors such as insurance status and ability to pay for care, and also in terms of biases that may influence health practitioners' diagnostic and treatment decisions.

Henry J. Kaiser Family Foundation (2004). The Uninsured: A Primer. People without health insurance make less use of needed medical services, are sicker when diagnosed with a medical problem, and die earlier. This report is a good background document to learn more about the importance of health insurance coverage.

Davis, K. et al. "Mirror, Mirror on the Wall: An Update on the Quality of American Health Care Through the Patient's Lens," The Commonwealth Fund, April 2006. This report is based on two surveys of patients: the first in 2004 among a nationally representative sample of adults in Australia, Canada, New Zealand, the United Kingdom, and the United States; the second conducted in 2005 among adults with health problems in the same five nations and Germany. The results of the surveys ranks patients' ratings of various dimensions of their health care, based on the Institute of Medicine's framework for quality assessment. The IOM quality domains included patient safety, effectiveness, patient-centeredness, timeliness, efficiency, and equity. Overall, the findings indicate that the U.S. health care system ranked first on clinical effectiveness, measured by levels of preventive care, care for the chronically ill, and hospital care, but ranked last on other dimensions of quality. Although these findings underscore the significant investment the United States makes in medical care delivery, it suggests that the U.S. could do much better in achieving high-quality health care for its population, particularly in light of the significantly higher per capita spending and continued disparities in terms of financial barriers to health care and access to services.

Gusmano, M. K. et al. "A New Way to Compare Health Systems: Avoidable Hospital Conditions in Manhattan and Paris." Health Affairs 25(2) (2006): 510–520. This study compares two similar large cities within two countries among the higher income countries of the Organization for Economic Cooperation and Development (OECD). Both cities are centers of medical excellence, and have similar per capita rates of physicians, acute hospital beds, and health outcomes as expressed by life expectancy years after the age of sixty-five. However, based on a comparison of hospital discharges for avoidable hospital conditions the authors found that Paris provides greater access to primary care than Manhattan. While rates of discharge for avoidable health conditions are higher among residents of low-income neighborhoods in both cities, the disparity among high- and low-income neighborhoods is more than twice as great in Manhattan. The authors conclude that the fact that the United States has no universal insurance coverage hinders access to timely, effective primary care, and, that even the presence of a strong health care safety net (as there is in Manhattan) does not substitute for health insurance coverage.

Infant Mortality

The David and Lucille Packard Foundation, The Future of Children— Low Birth Weight, Volume 5, Number 1 (1995). This group of articles looks at the rate and causes of low birth weight in the U.S., its relationship to infant mortality, and medical treatments to reduce the rate of infant death.

U.S. Department of Health and Human Services, Centers for Disease Control and Prevention, National Vital Statistics System, National Vital Statistics Reports, Volume 53, Number 5: Deaths: Final Data for 2002, October 14, 2004. This article discusses the socioeconomic differences in infant mortality and the ten leading causes of death for infants.

U.S. Department of Health and Human Services, Centers for Disease Control and Prevention, MMWR Weekly 54(22) (June 10, 2005): 553–556: Racial/Ethnic Disparities in Infant Mortality, U.S. 1995–2002. This article breaks down infant mortality rates by state/area of residence and the ethnicity of the mother.

U.S. Department of Health and Human Services, Centers for Disease Control and Prevention, Infant Mortality Fact Sheet: Eliminate Disparities in Infant Mortality, accessed at http://www.cdc.gov/omh/AMH/factsheets/ infant.htm. This fact sheet relates the differences in infant mortality rate and the leading causes of death between races. It also discusses the Healthy People 2010 campaign and the actions that public health agencies, medical care providers, and the community can take to improve behaviors that may affect infant mortality, such as smoking, substance abuse, and prenatal care.

Hessol N.A. and Fuentes-Afflick (2005). Ethnic Differences in Neonatal and Postneonatal Mortality, Pediatrics 115: 44–51. Updated information is available at http://www.pediatrics.org/cgi/content/full/115/1/e44. This article discusses the different rates of infant mortality among races and examines possible causes for these differences.

For more information about infant mortality and its determinants and consequences, see March of Dimes statistics website, Peristats, http://www .marchofdimes.com/peristats/default.aspx.

Medical Care

Cutler, David M. Your Money or Your Life. (2004). New York, Oxford University Press. In this book, David Cutler presents much of his previous research on the value of medical technology in extending survival and quality of life, and argues that the incremental benefits that patients receive clearly justify the costs. For example, since 1950, advances in heart disease treatment have brought a four-to-one return on each dollar spent by reducing the rate of death after heart attack by seventy-five percent and by extending survival to middle-aged Americans by three to five years. Despite the benefits of medical advancements, he suggests that we could produce the same level of improved health, in some cases, at lower costs, if we used medical technology more appropriately (used less overall) and coupled its use with lower cost healthy lifestyle changes. One example of this trade-off is encouraging smoking cessation programs for pregnant women since smoking during pregnancy is a large contributor to high-risk low-birth-weight babies and smoking cessation programs costs far less than neonatal intensive care services.

Hussey P. S., G. F. Anderson, R. Osborn, C. Feek, V. McLaughlin, Epstein A. Millar. How Does the Quality of Care Compare in Five Countries? Health Affairs 23(3) (2004): 89–99. Medical care is often measured by how well it performs in treating illness, delaying death, and in the satisfaction of patients who use physician and other medical services. This report studies the differences in health system outcomes among the United States, the United Kingdom, Canada, Australia, and New Zealand. No country consistently outperformed another country. The U.S. performed relatively well in several areas of medical care—breast cancer survival, cervical cancer screening rates, and shorter wait times for non-urgent surgery.

Gratzer, David. "Where Would You Rather Be Sick?" Wall Street Journal, June 15, 2006, page A14. This editorial disagrees with allegations that countries with a national health system (Canada, specifically) are healthier and have better access to health care than Americans, and at lower costs. The author acknowledges that Americans have higher rates of diabetes, arthritis, and high blood pressure, which he attributes to genetics, lifestyle, and culture rather than access to medical services. If we measure how well the U.S. health system serves its sick citizens, we do quite well: the mortality rate for prostate cancer is nineteen percent compared with twenty-five percent and fifty-seven percent in Canada and the United Kingdom, respectively. The author concludes by saying that our public health system needs improvement but our medical system, albeit expensive, provides timely access to needed medical care, particularly specialty services.

Blendon R., M. Kim, J. M. Benson. The Public Versus the World Health Organization on Health System Performance. Health Affairs 20(3) (May/June 2001): 10–20. This article takes issue with the World Health Organization's (WHO) report that ranked the U.S. lower than many countries on performance and citizen satisfaction, and disputes WHO's ranking of the health systems of 191 countries. The author claims that the WHO study fails to incorporate the level of satisfaction that the citizens feel towards their health system. In both cases, the United States scored low; however, the U.S. did rank number one in terms of responsiveness of its health care system, which may reflect a greater level of citizen satisfaction than indicated in the report.

CHAPTER 2

Is the United States So Different from Other Countries?

Anderson, Gerard F. et al. "It's the Price's, Stupid: Why the United States Is So Different Than Other Countries." Health Affairs 22(3) (May/June

2003). The United States spends more per capita on health care than any other developed country and has the greatest amount of privately funded health care. The United States has lower rates for hospital admissions and length of stay, but still has higher overall costs, which can be attributed to higher prices for supplies, equipment and drugs; more intensive treatment; and more generous payments to physicians.

Reinhart, Uwe, Peter S. Hussey and Gerard F. Anderson. "U.S. Health Care Spending in an International Context." Health Affairs (May/June 2004). The United States spends more on health care than twenty-nine other industrialized countries. Despite the fact that the U.S. has fewer nurses and physicians per capita, fewer hospital beds, and fewer imaging machines than many other countries, our overall spending is greater. The reasons for this increased spending include higher prices for services and labor, fewer ways to limit the supply of goods and services, greater administrative costs, and higher prescription drug prices. Price controls in other countries keep the price of labor and pharmaceuticals down compared with the U.S.

Anderson, Gerard F. et al. "Health Spending in the U.S. and the Rest of the Industrialized World." Health Affairs 24(4) (2005). The United States spends fifty-three percent more on health care than the rest of the industrialized world. The factors that increase cost include higher prices, more use of technology, an aging population, waste, inefficiency, the legal system, new disease patterns, and the U.S. health care market. Medical services in the U.S. are used with greater intensity. Even if the U.S. were to adopt similar supply restrictions and legal reforms found in other countries, the authors do not believe the U.S. would greatly reduce health care spending, because higher prices, incomes, and cost of living differences create the disparity between the U.S. and other developed countries.

Anderson, G.F. et al. "Health Care Spending and Use of Information Technology In OECD Countries." Health Affairs 25(3) (2006): 819–831. U.S. health care spending per capita was almost two and a half times the per capita health spending of the median Organization for Economic Cooperation and Development (OECD) country. Possible explanations for the higher spending include complex administrative "systems," increased use of invasive medical services, defensive medicine, lack of waiting lists, and higher prices for physician visits, hospital stays, and pharmaceuticals. The authors of this article explore how the use of health information technologies (HIT) has the potential for lowering spending and improving quality.

However, because of the fragmented nature of private/public U.S. medical care, (including problems of having systems that can share information, funding, and privacy concerns) adoption of HIT has been slow, and the United States now lags as much as a dozen years behind other countries in HIT adoption.

Iles, Andrew. "Spending on the UK Health Care Is Increasing Faster than Other Public Spending." BMJ 327 (2003). Demand for medical technologies increases health spending in all countries, and this article reports ways in which the United Kingdom, like the U.S., continues to spend a greater amount on health care over time. The National Health Service received seventeen percent of the total public spending in 2001–2002, which is the highest it has been since 1948. Health care spending in the U.K., as a part of GDP, lags behind other European countries, yet is growing at a faster rate than other components of its GDP, which suggests that the country will continue to spend more on health care.

Wilson, Jennifer Fisher. "Cheaper Drugs in Foreign Markets Increase the Focus on Domestic Drug Prices." American College of Physicians 2004. The United States pays more for prescription drugs than any other country, because we have not negotiated price controls with pharmaceutical companies. Drugs that are under patent are thirty to fifty percent more expensive in the U.S. than in other countries. However, generic drugs in the U.S. are often less expensive and more available than in other countries. Importation or re-importation of drugs from foreign countries may lower pharmaceutical prices and spending in the U.S., but the pharmaceutical industry will claim this reduction in payment will reduce new drug research and development.

The Reasons for Higher Medical Care Spending

Bozic, Kevin J. et al. "Health Care Technology Assessment. Basic Principles and Applications." The Journal of Bone and Joint Surgery 2004. Technological advances improve health outcomes and health care costs, but balancing the costs and benefits is necessary. The author believes that physicians can take an active part in preventing over-use of unnecessary procedures by learning about the importance of technology assessment during their medical training.

Pauly, Mark V. "Should We Be Worried about High Real Medical Spending Growth in the United States?" Health Affairs, January 8, 2003. Pauly tries to put the growth in health care spending, as a part of GDP, in perspective by explaining how GDP is influenced by consumers' preferences and the overall growth of GDP. The increase in medical spending and costs come from increased technological advances that have led to greater improvements in diagnosis and treatment of diseases, as well as in better health outcomes. He argues that these improvements in health may outweigh the costs of increased utilization of technology, but that technology assessment and eventual limitation may be needed to compensate for the possible overuse of technologies brought about as a result of consumer and provider demand.

Garber, Alan M. "Can Technology Assessment Control Health Spending?" *Health Affairs (Summer 1994), 116–126.* This article discusses technology assessment as a way to control the increasing costs of health care and to determine the effectiveness of little known procedures. The author suggests that, in the short run, insurance coverage has led to an overuse of technology and, in the long run, has influenced the development and distribution of the technology. Technology assessment can help determine whether new technologies substitute for older, less effective technologies, or whether new technologies complement existing technologies and increase the demand for both procedures, leading to increased overall spending.

Cutler, David M. and Mark McClellan. *"Is Technological Change in Medicine Worth It?" Health Affairs, September/October 2001.* The authors use five diseases to show how increased technology has improved the quality of life, productivity, and lifespan of people living with the disease. In four out of the five diseases, the authors found that the benefit generated from the increased quality of life outweighed the costs of the procedures. Cutler examines and amplifies his thesis in his book, *Your Money or Your Life: Strong Medicine for America's Health Care System* (NY: Oxford University Press, 2004). He suggests that we could produce the same level of health care benefits at even lower costs if we decreased overuse of advanced medical technologies.

Gratzer, D. *"The Return of HillaryCare: Socialized Medicine Is Still Not a Good Idea." The Weekly Standard, May 23, 2005, accessed through www .MedicalProgressToday.com (May 19, 2005).* The author states that the U.S. does receive value for the money it spends on medical care. He cites as evidence of the success of the U.S. health care system through comparisons with other European countries in the area of diagnosis and treatment of cancer. Specifically, he states that (according to Datamonitor and the World Health Organization) ninety-five percent of American women with breast cancer are diagnosed in early stages compared to less than eighty percent in Europe, and that survival rates for esophageal cancer and leukemia are almost twice as high in the United States.

Woolhandler, Steffie et al. "Costs of Health Care Administration in the U.S. and Canada." New England Journal of Medicine 349: 8 (2004). The United States spends thirty-one percent of its total health care costs on administration, compared with 16.7 percent in Canada, as a result of our fragmented system of private health care. The authors also suggest that U.S. administrative costs are high because of the greater need for utilization controls, accounting, and auditing.

Woolhandler, Steffie and David Himmelstein. "Costs of Care and Administration at For-profit and Other Hospitals in the U.S." New England Journal of Medicine 336(1) (1997). The authors report that for-profit hospitals spend more on hospital administration than non-profit hospitals. In 1994, for-profit hospitals used thirty-four percent of overall spending on administration, while non-profits spent 24.5 percent. This disparity suggests that for-profit hospital care is less efficient than in non-profit hospitals, despite for-profit hospitals' lower average length of stay.

CHAPTER 3

Too Much Medical Care

Wennberg, John E., Elliott S. Fisher, and Jonathan S. Skinner. "Geography and the Debate over Medicare Reform." Health Affairs Web Exclusive, February 13, 2002: W96-W114. This study examines Medicare spending across the country and finds that spending varies more than two times among regions with no improvement in health outcomes. Higher levels of increased Medicare spending are due mainly to increased use of physician visits, specialist consultations, and hospitalizations, particularly for those with chronic illnesses or in the last six months of life. It is this study that reported that, if spending levels in the lowest regions were realized in all higher regions, a savings of 28.9 percent would be realized. This has been widely interpreted and generalized as the U.S. "wasting one-third of medical dollars."

Wennberg, J. E. et al. "The Care of Patients with Severe Chronic Illness: A Report on the Medicare Program by the Dartmouth Atlas Project." (2006) The Center for the Evaluative Clinical Sciences, Dartmouth Medical School. This report analyzes the care given to the Medicare population for severe chronic illnesses such as diabetes, heart disease, and cancer, and looks at the differences in spending across regions of the United States. The authors found that chronically ill patients living in high spending regions have more visits, hospitalizations, intensive care unit stays, and more diagnostic tests, with no accompanying benefit in length or quality of life. In fact, those with chronic illnesses who live in regions that spend more have slightly shorter life expectancies and less satisfaction with their care than those living in regions with lower rates of spending. The authors conclude that Medicare spending could be reduced by thirty percent if the use of resources were kept to the level of the more efficient regional providers.

What Do We Mean by Waste?

Phillips, Robert L. et al. "Can Nurse Practitioners and Physicians Beat Parochialism into Plowshares?" Health Affairs 21(5) (2002): 133–142. In recent years, what nurse practitioners are permitted to do has expanded greatly, and advanced practice nurses in general may now share some of the same duties as physicians. Studies have shown that collaboration between nurse practitioners and physicians increases quality of care, improves physician job satisfaction, reduces overall workload, and suggests that nurse practitioner-physician teams will be part of a more efficient health care system.

Miller, Tracy E. and Arthur R. Derse. "Between Strangers: The Practice of Medicine Online." Health Affairs, July/August 2002: 168–179. This article discusses the benefits and problems with the new practice of online medicine. Online medicine, or the electronic interaction between a patient and a physician, may improve the quality of health care and deliver care in a more timely way. In 2001, about three million people sought advice for a specific medical condition online. People can join disease management programs, obtain second opinions online, or e-mail their physician. Concerns about online medicine include patient privacy, and the absence of face-to-face interaction. Policy makers need to define the boundaries of online medicine, and establish physician accountability and fair reimbursement policies.

Assessing "Waste" in Medical Care

"Medicare Definition of Fraud." Center for Medicare and Medicaid Services. The Center for Medicare and Medicaid Services (CMS) oversees the two largest federal programs for medical care, Medicare and Medicaid. This document defines fraud as a misrepresentation or false statement about the payment owed to a supplier, employer, billing service, patient, or institution. Violations include billing for fraudulent diagnoses and for services that were never performed, and falsifying records

"Fighting Fraud, Waste, and Abuse in Medicare and Medicaid." Center for Medicare and Medicaid Services. February 22, 1999. Efforts such as Operation Restore Trust have reduced waste, fraud, and abuse in Medicare and Medicaid, and have recovered $1.2 billion dollars over the past two years. Under Operation Restore Trust, every dollar spent to identify abuse recovered $23 in funds judged to be "misused." Other initiatives, such as Medicare Integrity Program, helped to reduce overpayments and errors in Medicare and Medicaid billing.

"The Medicare Integrity Program: Pay it Right!" Health Care Financing Administration. March Publication No. HCFA-02201, March 2001. In 1996, the Medicare Integrity Program (MIP) was formed to improve efficiency in cost reporting, auditing, medical review, and anti-fraud in Medicare administration. In 1996, fourteen percent of Medicare payments were said to be made improperly. After implementation of MIP, errors in payments were reduced to 7.8 percent. In 1997, Medicare's administrator said that the most common mistake in payments was paying for unnecessary medical care.

Mitchell, Colby L. et al. "Billing for Inpatient Hospital Care." American Society of Health-System Pharmacists 60(6) (2003). This article discusses the importance of accurate documentation and billing for payment and to protect hospitals from lawsuits. It describes the different forms used for billing and the types of hospital charges.

Thorpe, Kenneth. "Inside the Black Box of Administrative Costs." Health Affairs, Summer 1992: 42–55. The U.S. has higher administrative costs because of its fragmented public/private payer medical "system"; as well, health systems in the United States have broader objectives, such as collecting clinical data to improve the delivery of medical care and investing in information and data processing systems, all of which add to administrative costs, but may reduce health care spending over the long term. The author argues it is difficult to compare our costs with other countries that have a single administrative system.

Woolhandler, Steffie, Terry Campbell and David U. Himmelstein. "Health Care Administration in the United States and Canada: Micromanagement, Macro Costs." International Journal of Health Services 34.1 (2004): 65–78. This article compares the amount spent on administrative costs between the U.S. and Canada and suggests reasons why the U.S. has a greater amount of money devoted to health care administration (thirty-one percent of medical care spending in the U.S. compared with 16.7 percent in Canada). Functions essential in private insurance, such as advertising as well as determining medical risk to price the insurance premium, are absent in public systems such as Canada's, and account for about two-thirds of the private insurers' administrative costs. The authors believe that America's fragmented payment system and the private insurance market may be reasons that the U.S. devotes a greater proportion of health care spending to administrative costs, and that reducing U.S. administrative costs to Canadian levels could save at least $290 billion annually.

Bodenheimer, Thomas. "The Not-So-Sad History of Medicare Cost Containment as Told in One Chart." Health Affairs 23 (January 2003): W33-W90. Medicare expenditures per enrollee have decreased while overall U.S. expenditures for medical care have increased. Medicare growth is estimated at six percent, while private insurance companies grew at 11.5 percent. The author suggests cost-containment measures, such as reducing administrative costs and unnecessary medical treatments, which could curb the increased growth rate of health expenditures.

Bodenheimer, Thomas and Alicia Fernandez. "High and Rising Health Care Costs. Part 4: Can Costs Be Controlled by Preserving Quality?" Annals of Internal Medicine 143(1) (2005): 26–32. The authors believe that physicians play a large role in helping to regulate how quickly technology (such as a new drug or device) gets used and which services are performed. If technology is used quickly and services increase, the overall cost of medical care increases. In terms of patients, focus should be aimed at high-cost, frequent users of health care services since seventy percent of all health expenditures are concentrated in ten percent of the population. The authors cite several examples of inappropriate medical care, and note that high-intensity care often does not translate into better health outcomes. The authors believe that shared decision making between doctor and patient as well as better technology assessment will help reduce inappropriate care and medical expenses.

Menzel, Paul et al. "Toward a Broader View of Values in Cost-Effectiveness Analysis of Health." Hastings Center Report, May–June 1999: 7–15. This article explores how individual preferences that reflect overall "intangible" societal values might be better incorporated into the "effectiveness" side of cost-effectiveness analysis (CEA) when making allocation decisions. The authors suggest that, in addition to quantitatively measuring specific benefits of medical treatments, cost-effectiveness analysis should be broadened to include some of the more intangible values such as preserving the hope for treatment for those who are seriously ill in the face of death. Although inefficient by CEA standards, these types of ethical considerations reflect a larger societal utility and should be considered in how we decide what is important and "effective" in deciding which medical care treatments are worthwhile.

Garber, Alan M. "Cost-effectiveness and Evidence Evaluation as Criteria for Coverage Policy." Health Affairs 19 (May 2004). Garber explains the importance of addressing the problem of rising health care costs by examining which procedures are offered by health insurance plans. Currently, health insurance covers "medically necessary" procedures, but the high rate of innovation in medical products and services presumably leads to better health, but also higher spending. Garber believes that to contain costs, health plans need to weigh the benefits of procedures with the costs, and how cost-effectiveness analysis could be better used in health insurance coverage decisions.

Neumann, Peter J. and Magnus Johannesson. "From Principle to Public Policy: Using Cost-Effectiveness Analysis." Health Affairs (Summer 1994): 207–214. This article discusses cost-effectiveness analysis, the problems and issues associated with it, and the ways in which it is being used to decide what medical care to pay for. The author believes that cost-effectiveness analysis is a worthy goal, but that using it in health coverage decisions has been difficult because of the problems in measuring patient preferences and quality of life. The article looks at how different public payers in the United States (such as Medicare) and other countries address these issues.

CHAPTER 4

Calfo, S. et al. "Last Year of Life Study." Office of the Actuary, Centers for Medicare and Medicaid Services. This federal agency reports the costs for Medicare enrollees who died in 1999 were averaged $24,856 per person compared with survivor costs of $3,669. These statistics and this study was also cited in the Kaiser Family Foundation Medicare Chartbook, 3rd edition, summer 2005, accessed at http://www.kff.org/medicare/7284.cfm.

Emanuel, Ezekiel J. and Linda L. Emanuel. "The Economics of Dying—The Illusion of Cost Savings at the End of Life." New England Journal of Medicine 330(8) (1994): 540–544. This article summarizes the high cost of medical care associated with end-of-life treatment and examines the role of advance directives, hospice, and futile care in achieving cost savings. Two million Americans die each year, accounting for about ten to twelve percent of health care expenditures. Medicare patients who die in any given year spend up to seven times more on medical care than an average Medicare patient. The authors suggest that advance directives will not decrease overall medical costs because patients often request more life-sustaining treatment, eliminating any cost savings; while hospice can reduce medical costs, the longer the person stays in hospice, the fewer saving there will be. The authors conclude that there is not much money to be saved at the end of life, and that the amount that might be saved by reducing the use of aggressive life-sustaining treatments such as "Do Not Resuscitate" (DNR) orders, or increasing the use of advance directives or hospice care will save at most six percent of Medicare expenditures and 3.3 percent of the total national health care expenditures.

Scitovsky, Anne A. "The High Cost of Dying Revisited." The Milbank Quarterly 72(4) (1994): 561–591. This article examines the high cost of end-of-life elderly care, and supports earlier studies that showed that medical care costs in the last year of life are high, and that elderly Medicare patients who are dying account for a high proportion of total Medicare expenditures. The author concludes that advance directives, hospice, and DNR orders do not necessarily decrease the cost or use of unnecessary end-of-life procedures, and suggests that a closer patient-physician relationship and a change in Americans' expectations of what medical care can accomplish would be more effective at controlling costs at the end of life.

Kramer, Andrew M. "Health Care for Elderly Persons—Myths and Realities." New England Journal of Medicine 332(15) (1995): 1027–1029. This editorial discusses the difference in end-of-life treatment and costs by age, and suggests that the older the person is, the less expensive the yearly cost of care. The author states that hospice, advance directives, and less intensive treatment reduce health expenditures by only three percent, confirming earlier studies. He suggests that there may be opportunities for greater savings if advanced directives and DNR orders are put in place by patients when they are young before a crisis occurs. In addition, the author suggests that additional cost savings may be possible if there was a greater emphasis on keeping the elderly healthy and avoiding hospitalization

Emanuel, Ezekiel J. "Cost Savings at the End of Life: What Do the Data Show?" JAMA 275(24) (1996): 1907–1914. This commentary argues against the commonly held belief that increased use of hospice and advance directives and lower use of interventions for terminally ill patients will produce significant cost savings at the end of life. He reports that existing data suggest that hospice and advance directives can save ten to seventeen percent in the last six months of life and zero to ten percent in the last year of life. Even so, the author cautions us not to discount the value of hospice and advance directives because, while they may not achieve huge medical savings at the end of life, they nevertheless may have additional value for patients if they reflect patient preferences for care.

Hogan, Christopher, June Lunney, Jon Gabel, and Joanne Lynn. "Medicare Beneficiaries' Costs of Care in the Last Year of Life." Health Affairs 20(4) (2001). This article discusses the cost of care in the last year of life for Medicare patients. More than one-quarter of Medicare payments are for the last year of life, unchanged from twenty years ago. The authors believe that high end-of-life care is not a significant cost driver because the percentage Medicare devotes to care at the end of life has remained stable. The authors believe that much of what has been labeled "the high cost of dying" is the cost of caring for severe illness, whether someone is dying or not.

Teno, Joan M. "Advance Directives for Nursing Home Residents: Achieving Compassionate, Competent, Cost-effective Care." JAMA 283(11) (2000): 1481–1482. This editorial discusses the role of advance directives in reducing medical costs for nursing home residents by reducing hospital admissions from the nursing home, for a savings of $1,200 per patient. The author believes that nursing home care will play an increasingly important role in the care of the dying since the proportion of deaths occurring in nursing homes is expected to increase to forty percent over the next fifteen years.

As such, the use of advance directives for the nursing home population may help control costs at the end of life.

Levinsky, Norman G. et al. "Influence of Age on Medicare Expenditures and Medical Care in the Last Year of Life." JAMA 286(11) (2001). This article examines the effects of age on medical spending and the amount of end-of-life treatment. The study found that the cost of care decreases as age increases in both hospice care and other care. The cost of inpatient end-of-life care was greater than nursing home and residential care. The use of the intensive care unit as well as intensive medical and surgical procedures all decreased as age increased, suggesting that physicians are more likely to treat younger patients more intensely.

Huskamp, Haiden A., Melinda Beeuwkes Buntin, Virginia Wang, and Joseph P. Newhouse. "Providing Care at the End of Life: Do Medicare Rules Impede Good Care?" Health Affairs 20(3) (2001). The authors make recommendations for changes in Medicare that would encourage the use of hospice and home health services. For example, Medicare requires that for a physician to order "hospice care" the patient must be expected to die within six months. Physicians may not refer patients to hospice because they are uncertain if the patient will die within six months. If the patient does not die within the allotted hospice time, then the physician could face charges of fraud. The authors assessed problems faced by several types of providers delivering end-of-life services, and identified ways to improve Medicare coverage at the end of life.

Buntin, Melinda Beeuwkes and Haiden Huskamp. "What Is Known about the Economics of End-of-Life Care for Medicare Beneficiaries?" The Gerontologist. 42(3) (2002): 40–48. This article discusses differences in end-of-life care for elderly patients in hospitals, nursing homes, and hospice care. It also discusses the variation in quality of care among these providers, partly as a result of the different billing practices and policies. The study discusses the racial and socioeconomic disparities, practices, and reasons for end-of-life care. For example, African Americans use twenty-five percent less care in the three years before death than white persons, but eighteen percent more in the last year of life, mostly as a result of inpatient care. The authors state that barriers to the use of hospice by minority populations are distrust of the medical system and a preference to die in the hospital. It also discusses the responsibility of physicians to discuss end-of-life decisions and give realistic estimates of time left to live. Medicare spending on end-of-life care has been constant for decades. The greater the supply of hospice services in a geographic region of the United States, the longer the length of stay in hospice before death. A 1996 Gallup Poll found that ninety percent of people said they would prefer to die in their home if they had six months to live. Physicians and patients overestimate the probability of survival, which influences treatment decisions and encourages life-extending care over "comfort care."

Emanuel Ezekiel J., Arlene Ash, Wei Yu, Gail Gazelle, Norman G. Levinsky, Olga Saynina, Mark McClellan, Mark Moskowitz. Managed Care, Hospice Use, Site of Death, and Medical Expenditures in the Last Year of Life. Archives of Internal Medicine 162 (August 12–26, 2002). The article examines deaths of Medicare beneficiaries in Massachusetts and California to evaluate the effect of managed care on the use of hospice, and to determine how hospice affects the expenditures for the last year of life. There has been increasing concern about the high costs of end-of-life care, estimated to be five times the expenditures for the average Medicare beneficiary, and the hope that hospice could reduce such costs. The authors found that those who died and were covered by Medicare in California were more likely to be enrolled in managed care organizations, were more likely to use a hospice, and had lower hospitalization rates than those in Massachusetts, yet there were few differences in expenditures in the last year of life: $27,814 per person who died per year in California and $28,588 per person in Massachusetts.

Campbell, Diane E. et al. "Medicare Program Expenditures Associated with Hospice Use." Annals of Internal Medicine 140(4) (2004): 269–278. Between the years of 1992 and 2000, the total number of patients in hospice increased by fourteen percent, with cancer patients in hospice care increasing by twenty-five percent. The study claims that for people without cancer or who are older than eighty, hospice care actually has few or no cost savings because of the constant services of hospice care. Expenditures were four percent higher overall among hospice patients compared with those not in hospice, and eleven percent higher for hospice patients without cancer. Savings were highest (seven to seventeen percent) for hospice enrollees with lung and other very aggressive types of cancer diagnosed in the last year of life.

Barnato, Amber E., Mark B. McClellan, Christopher R. Kagay, and Alan M. Garber. "Trends in Inpatient Treatment Intensity among Medicare Ben-

eficiaries at the End of Life." Health Services Research 39(2) (2004). The proportion of total Medicare expenditures for care in the last year of life (approximately thirty percent to the five percent of Medicare patients who die each year) has not declined over the last two decades. This study suggests that despite the fact that there has been a decline in in-hospital deaths for Medicare patients, there has not been a decrease in per capita utilization of expensive inpatient services in the last year of life. We are doing more intensive treatment of all Medicare beneficiaries when they enter the hospital, even for those who are at the end of life, despite the fact that much of this medical care is futile.

Hampson, Lindsay A. and Ezekiel J. Emanuel. "The Prognosis for Change in End-of-Life Care After the Schiavo Case." Health Affairs 24(4) (2005): 972–975. This article summarizes the effect that the Terri Schiavo case had on the public and on political views of end-of-life treatment, and suggests that we will continue to see cases where efforts to terminate futile care for dying patients will meet resistance from patients' families. The article reports that only twenty percent of Americans have completed living wills and that family members are poor at predicting patients' wishes for life-sustaining treatment.

St. John, Elaine B., Kathleen G. Nelson, Suzanne P. Cliver, Rita R. Bishnoi, Robert L. Goldenberg. "Cost of Neonatal Care According to Gestational Age at Birth and Survival Status." American Journal of Obstetrics and Gynecology, 182(1.1) (January 2000): 170–175. This study examined the cost of initial hospital care for newborn infants. The authors found that length of stay and age of the newborn were related to cost among survivors born at less than or at thirty-two weeks' gestation. Total cost of initial care of the U.S. population of newborns is estimated at $10.2 billion annually, with 11.9 percent spent on infants born between twenty-four and twenty-six weeks of age and 42.7 percent spent on those born at thirty-seven weeks or later.

Gilbert William M., Thomas S. Nesbitt, Beate Danielsen. "The Cost of Prematurity: "Quantification by Gestational Age and Birth Weight." Obstetrics & Gynecology 102(3) (September 2003): 488–492. This article looks at how pregnancy outcomes and costs were associated with prematurity in surviving infants. Hospital costs for preterm babies averaged $202,700 for a delivery at twenty-five weeks, decreasing to $2,600 for a thirty-six-week newborn and $1,100 for a thirty-eight-week newborn, with total costs of $38 million dollars for each preterm newborn age group from twenty-five to thirty-six weeks. The authors conclude that prematurity is associated with significant neonatal hospital costs, all of which decrease as infants are born closer to full term.

Hack Maureen, Taylor H. Gerry, Dennis Drotar, Mark Schluchter, Lydia Cartar, Laura Andreias, Deanne Wilson-Costello, Nancy Klein. "Chronic Conditions, Functional Limitations, and Special Health Care Needs of School-aged Children Born with Extremely Low Birth Weight in the 1990s." JAMA 294(3) (2005): 318–325. This article examines school-age functioning and special health care needs of extremely-low-birth-weight (ELBW) children (less than 1,000 grams or about two pounds) and compared these children with normal-birth-weight children. The authors found that eight years after birth, sixty-five percent of ELBW children had significantly more chronic conditions than normal birth-weight children, including cerebral palsy, vision problems, lower IQ, limited academic skills, and poor motor skills. The authors suggest that ELBW infants who survive into child- and adulthood have considerable long-term health and educational needs.

U.S. Department of Health and Human Services, "Criteria for Determining Disability in Infants and Children: Low Birth Weight." Agency for Health Care Quality (AHRQ) Evidence Report/Technology Assessment No. 70, Pub. No. 03-E008, 2002. This report examines the evidence that premature infants born weighing less than three pounds with or without other conditions is associated with long-term disabling outcomes. The primary disabilities discussed in this report are cerebral palsy, mental retardation, hearing/speech/language/behavioral problems, vision problems, lung problems, and problems with growth. Findings report that over half of premature infants have disabilities, often severe, and that long-term complications result in significant costs to the family and society for medical care.

For additional easy-to-read consumer information on the costs of premature infant care, see: *"The Big Picture: Hospital Costs," March of Dimes Birth Defects Foundation (2005), available at: http://www.marchofdimes.com/prematurity.* This fact sheet profiles the costs associated with premature infant care compared with that of a healthy baby. Nearly half of the total 2002 hospital charges for infants, $15.5 billion out of $33.8 billion, were for small and/or premature babies.

CHAPTER 5

Doing the Right Things "Right"

McGlynn, Elizabeth A. et al. "The Quality of Health Care Delivered to Adults in the United States." New England Journal of Medicine 348(26) (2003): 2635–2645. Individuals in this study were asked about their health care experiences in order to evaluate if their care was consistent with basic quality standards regarding the use of preventive, chronic, and acute medical care. "Recommended care" was decided by a panel of experts based on national guidelines taken from the medical literature. Examples of conditions surveyed included alcohol dependence, asthma, breast cancer, colorectal cancer, and coronary artery (heart) disease. The study found the following: (1) a little more than half of the participants (54.9 percent) received care felt by the experts to be appropriate, i.e., "recommended care"; (2) 54.9 percent received recommended preventive care; (3) 53.5 percent received recommended acute care; (4) 56.1 percent received recommended chronic care; (5) 52.2 percent received screenings; and (6) 58.5 percent received recommended follow-up care. The authors also found that 46.3 percent received less than they should have ("underuse") and 11.3 percent received more than they should have ("overuse"). These results expose a real quality gap between what we know to be important in improving health care and actually delivering that care to adults in the United States.

Institute of Medicine, "Crossing the Quality Chasm: A New Health System for the 21st Century." March 2001 (http://www.iom.edu) . This Institute of Medicine (IOM) report sets goals to improve the quality of U.S. health care. These six goals include delivering safe, effective, patient-centered, timely, efficient and equitable care. The report outlines ten simple rules, or general principles, to help ensure that the health system is responsive and reduces risk to patients, including care that: is continuous in order to promote healing relationships; is customized according to patient needs and values; has the patient in control over health decisions; is based on the best scientific evidence; is delivered within a system of safety and with information that is understandable and geared toward patient satisfaction; anticipates patient needs; reduces waste of resources or patient time; and promotes cooperation, communication, and coordination among clinicians and health care services. In addition, the report calls for the private and public sectors to collaborate to analyze medical evidence, create practice guidelines, and develop a consistent way to evaluate quality of care. The IOM also recommends using computers to communicate with patients, to order prescriptions online, and to send reminders to patients and physicians about necessary medical care.

Berwick, Donald M. "A User's Manual for the IOM's 'Quality Chasm' Report." Health Affairs 21(3) (2002): 80–90. In this report, Berwick, a contributor to the Institute of Medicine (IOM) report above, simplifies that report. The IOM report identifies areas of misuse, overuse, and underuse of health care that contribute to the "quality chasm." He breaks down the improvements for reform by focusing on patients, health systems, and needed health policy. Berwick says that we need to develop a system that supports physician best practices, develop better information technology to distribute information and improve clinical decision making, and we need to use electronic health records and increased coordination of care. To accomplish these goals, the U.S. may need to develop incentives to encourage adoption of technology and changes in practice patterns.

Delivering High Quality Care May Be Expensive

National Institute for Health Care Management. "Prescription Drug Expenditures in 2001." Revised May 6, 2002. The report says that drugs that reduce cholesterol accounted for $10 billion in drug expenditures in 2001. For all drugs, anti-depressants were the highest expense, followed by those that lower cholesterol and then ulcer drugs.

Benner Joshua A., Robert J. Glynn, Helen Mogun, Peter J. Neumann, Milton C. Weinstein, and Jerry Avorn. "Long-term Persistence in Use of Statin Therapy in Elderly Patients." JAMA 288(4) (2002): 455–461. This study shows that the adherence rate in older patients for the appropriate use of lipid-lowering (statin) therapy to reduce heart disease and early death decreased over time. The proportion of patients who took their statin therapy correctly was sixty percent after three months, forty-three percent after six months, and twenty-six percent after five years.

Jackevicius Cynthia A., Muhammad Mamdani, Jack V. Tu. "Adherence With Statin Therapy in Elderly Patients With and Without Acute Coronary Syndromes." JAMA 288(4) (2002): 462–467. The study compares three groups of patients who had been prescribed drugs that lower lipids (statins): those who had severe chest pain or a heart attack in the last year; patients who had evidence of chronic heart disease; and those who had no heart disease. The authors found that, after two years of follow-up, only forty percent of patients in the chest pain/heart attack group, thirty-six percent in the group with known heart disease, and twenty-five percent in the group with no known heart disease were still taking statins. Although those most healthy took statins the least, in none of the groups did more than half of the patients take their medications as prescribed. Since the patients in this study were Canadian and the cost of the drugs carried only a $2 co-pay, expense should not have been part of the decision to stop taking the prescribed medication. The authors conclude that elderly patients with and without heart disease have low rates of continuing lipid-lowering drugs over time.

   Hillestad, Richard et al. "Can Electronic Medical Record Systems Transform Health Care? Potential Health Benefits, Savings, and Costs." Health Affairs 24(5) (2005): 1103–1117. This article examines the benefits and costs of electronic medical records (EMR) and their effects on health care expenditures. According to the authors, it is widely believed that EMR systems will lead to major health care savings, reduce medical errors, and improve health. However, in the U.S., EMR systems are not widely used due to the high costs of start-up, lack of standards, and differences between who pays and who benefits. The study suggests that effective EMR implementation and networking could save more than $81 billion annually by improving efficiency and safety, particularly in the areas of reducing hospital lengths of stay, nurses' administrative time, drug usage in hospitals, and radiology usage in the outpatient setting.

   Walker, James M. "Electronic Medical Records and Health Care Transformation." Health Affairs (September/October 2005): 1118–1120. In this article, the author's institution, Geisinger Clinic, has already implemented an EMR system and has had great success. However, the author is concerned that not all hospitals will be able to change their routines and procedures to be compatible with EMR processes because EMRs are so expensive to develop, integrate with existing systems, and then support. Despite the critical contribution EMR systems can make, the author concludes that the current state of the industry is too immature to predict the clinical benefits or cost savings of EMR systems.

   Goodman, Clifford. "Savings in Electronic Medical Record Systems? Do it for the Quality." Health Affairs 24(5) (2005): 1124–1126. The prospect of

EMR systems to decrease health costs is a potential selling point for investment in such systems but it is unclear, according to this author, that any real savings will significantly reduce overall health care spending. Nevertheless, the potential of EMRs and other types of health information technologies offer a direct means of addressing the quality deficits in the U.S. health care system and therefore should be pursued through governmental and private support to enable new forms of integrated health data collection, analysis, and knowledge development.

Miller, Robert H. "The Value of Electronic Health Records in Solo or Small Group Practices." Health Affairs 24(5) (2005): 1127–1137. This study examines the costs associated with the adoption of electronic medical records by small or individual group practices. The costs will determine how fast and how many physicians will use electronic medical records. Electronic medical systems can be used to write notes about patient visits, prescribe medications, and assist in billing. After implementation of the EMR, the medical groups realized cost savings as a result of billing efficiency and increased patient visits. Some physicians had difficulties with start-up, which reduced their efficiency and actually increased costs in the short term. However, those doctors who were successful working with EMRs experienced benefits including better patient records, less time spent creating records, and fewer mistakes in billing.

Fireman, Bruce, Joan Bartlett, and Joe Selby. "Can Disease Management Reduce Health Care Costs by Improving Quality?" Health Affairs 23(6) (2004): 63–75. Disease management programs allow patients to be active partners in managing their health, particularly if they receive treatment for many medical conditions. Through the use of a care manager, patients learn how to maintain their health, which means fewer visits to the emergency room and timely discharge from the hospital. Many payers are looking at disease management programs as a way to improve quality and reduce costs of health care. Those responsible for paying for medical care (government, employers, insurance companies) hope that disease management programs will help patients comply with medical care instructions, which in turn may reduce expensive hospital admissions and other medical costs. Programs using a disease management model include the use of clinical guidelines, patient education tools for self-management, disease registries, and community outreach. Some health plans utilize disease management programs for patients with coronary artery disease, heart failure, diabetes, and asthma.

The authors found that patients who were enrolled in disease management programs followed doctors' directions more often and reduced both blood pressure and cholesterol levels; however, costs increased. The study suggests that disease management programs have the potential to increase quality of care, and increase efficiency, but may not reduce costs.

Bodenheimer, Thomas and Alicia Fernandez. *"High and Rising Health Care Costs. Part 4: Can Costs Be Controlled While Preserving Quality?"* Annals of Internal Medicine 143(1) (2005): 26–32. In this article, the author describes a program run by nurses for patients after they are discharged from the hospital with congestive heart failure that reduced hospital readmissions, costs, and improved the patients' quality of life. Patient education programs also reduced hospital readmissions. While management programs have the potential to save money for those heavy users of health care resources, it would most likely increase overall health care costs if targeted to all patients with heart disease.

CHAPTER 6

Prevention Is Expensive

Shenkin, Henry. *"Is an Ounce of Prevention always Worth a Pound of Cure?"* Western Journal of Medicine 2001: 174–85. Shenkin states that it makes no sense to say that prevention will contain costs because screening large numbers of healthy people to find the few that will develop the specific disease costs more than it saves. He says that even if disease-prevention measures save money in the short term, the long-term costs will be greater as those persons develop expensive chronic illnesses in old age. The true value of preventive services lies in improving quality of life and longevity.

Barendregt, Jan J. et al. *"The Health Care Cost of Smoking."* New England Journal of Medicine 33(15) (1997): 1052–1057. In 1992, the Surgeon General said that smokers spend $6,000 more, on average, over a lifetime, on medical care than non-smokers. Smokers have greater per-person medical costs than non-smokers, but they often have a shorter life expectancy than non-smokers who will use a great amount of resources in their later years. Smokers use up to forty percent more medical services while they are alive, but the overall costs to society are four to seven percent less because smokers die earlier. Therefore, decreased smoking produced savings in the short run but increased costs in the long run.

Weinstein, Milton C. "The Costs of Prevention." J Gen Intern Med 5 (September/October Supplement, 1990): S89–92. This landmark article discusses the cost-effectiveness of prevention programs and analyzes the costs of prevention and care for the disease, and the costs and savings attributable to life extension. The author concludes that prevention does not usually save money except in certain specific cases such as water fluoridation or childhood vaccinations, that preventive interventions can be less expensive ways to buy healthy years of life than some medical treatments (but not always), and that prevention is more cost-effective when it can be incorporated into personal lifestyles rather than added on as a medical expense (e.g., physical activity and weight control rather than drugs for high blood pressure). The author argues that it is unrealistic to believe that prevention will "make" money for our health care system, but it may save lives and improve health.

The Costs of High Blood Pressure Treatment

Whelton Paul K., Jiang He, Lawrence J. Appel, Jeffrey A. Cutler, Stephen Havas, Theodore A. Kotchen, Edward J. Roccella, Ron Stout, Carlos Vallbona, Mary C. Winston, Joanne Karimbakas. "Primary Prevention of Hypertension: Clinical and Public Health Advisory from the National High Blood Pressure Education Program." JAMA 288(15) (2002): 1882–1888. This article discusses prevention strategies for forty-three million U.S. adults who have high blood pressure, and reports that approximately twenty million were not being treated with medication, and that twelve million of the nearly twenty-three million for whom medication was prescribed had poorly controlled high blood pressure. The authors suggest a primary prevention strategy that includes physical activity, dietary changes, and behavioral changes.

Frazier, Howard S. and Frederick Mosteller. Medicine Worth Paying For. Harvard University Press. Cambridge, Massachusetts: 1995. Chapter 10. The authors address the cost-effectiveness of hypertension treatment, and find that hypertension treatment does not pay for itself in savings in terms of the medical costs of strokes or heart attacks prevented. It recommends shifting resources away from prevention in younger populations to treating a targeted elderly population to increase the overall cost savings of high blood pressure treatment. This section also addresses policy issues and the effects of treatment on life expectancy and illness, and suggests that life expectancy change due to the elimination of hypertension would produce a gain of ten years from birth.

The Costs of Diabetes Treatment

The CDC Diabetes Cost-Effectiveness Group. "Cost-Effectiveness of Intensive Glycemic Control, Intensified Hypertension Control, and Serum Cholesterol Level Reduction for Type II Diabetes." JAMA 287(19) (2002): 2542–2550. The authors examine the cost and effectiveness of treatment for hypertension and the control of diabetes. High blood pressure control for the sickest patients was the only treatment to be found cost-effective. The other treatments all increased life-expectancy and improved health, but increased overall costs. Since treated patients often live longer, they may develop other diseases or complications that will also increase health costs.

Brown, Jonathan B., Kathryn L. Pedula, Alan W. Bakst. "The Progressive Cost of Complications in Type 2 Diabetes Mellitus." Archives of Internal Medicine 159 (1999): 1873–1880. This article looks at the costs of treating the long-term complications of diabetes. The authors found that per-person yearly costs increased by $1,087 for prevention of heart disease compared with a cost of $7,352 in treatment costs after a major cardiovascular event such as a heart attack or a stroke. The additional cost of care associated with kidney disease was similar—about $1,300 above baseline, which rose to $4,000 with the development of advanced kidney problems and up to $15,700 with the onset of treating kidney failure.

American Diabetes Association, "Direct and Indirect Costs of Diabetes in the United States," accessed at http://www.diabetes.org/diabetes-statistics/cost-of-diabetes-in-us.jsp. This fact sheet estimates the total economic cost of diabetes in 2002 to be $132 billion, with direct costs of diabetes of $92 billion, of which cardiovascular disease accounted for almost $18 billion of the annual direct medical costs. Indirect costs resulting from lost workdays, restricted activity days, mortality, and permanent disability due to diabetes totaled $40 billion.

U.S. Department of Health and Human Services, Centers for Disease Control and Prevention, National Center for Health Statistics. "U.S. Decennial

Life Tables for 1989–91." Volume 1, Number 4, DHHS Publication No. PHS-99-1150-4 (September 1999). This set of tables reports that the gain in life years for hypertension, diabetes, and leukemia is 9.56 years, 12.24 years, and 15.02 years, respectively.

Measles Vaccination

Frazier, Howard S. and Frederick Mosteller. Medicine Worth Paying For. Harvard University Press. Cambridge, Massachusetts: 1995. Chapter 9 in this book addresses measles and the cost savings of measles vaccinations. The vaccine is ninety-five percent effective and decreased the incidence of the disease by 99.8 percent from the year of licensing (1963) through 1982, with an estimated total savings of $5 billion dollars..

Lieu, Tracy A. et al. "Overcoming the Economic Barriers to the Optimal Use of Vaccines." Health Affairs (May/June 2005): 666–679. Vaccines are the most cost-effective form of health care intervention because some result in net savings. The cost of health care increases when schools or government require additional and new childhood vaccinations that may not be as cost-effective.

Homer, C. J. et al. "Does Quality of Care Affect Rates of Hospitalization for Childhood Asthma?" Pediatrics 98(1) (1996): 18–23. This article finds that preventive care in outpatients for childhood asthma decreases the hospitalization rate. The author concludes that preventive therapies play a key role in determining community hospitalization rates for chronic conditions such as childhood asthma.

Is There a Business Case for Prevention? Whose Dollars?

Leatherman, Sheila. "The Business Case for Quality: Case Studies and an Analysis." Health Affairs 22(2) (2003): 17–30. The business case for quality says that a business or provider that invests in preventive medical care will gain an increase in worker productivity and profits, and may have other benefits such as decreased hospitalization rates, which actually save money. A case study regarding a diabetes disease management program had higher costs in the short run but was predicted to save overall costs in the long run if patients remained in the program for a ten-year period. The authors conclude that preventive programs can have positive effects on both patients' and society's health, but in a fragmented health system where patients move among employers, practitioners, and health plans, it is often difficult to align incentives that promote quality improvement. Problems within the employment marketplace, such as high employee turnover, hindered the success of longer-term disease management programs to demonstrative improved outcomes as a result of preventive care.

National Business Group on Health, "Improving Health. Improving Business." Washington, DC (2005). Employers are dependent upon a healthy workforce to maintain maximum productivity. On an annual basis, $33 billion in medical costs and $9 billion in lost productivity because of heart disease, cancer, stroke, and diabetes is related to poor nutrition. Cardiovascular disease alone results in costs up to $150 billion in lost productivity. The report suggests that workplace-sponsored prevention services have the potential to improve health and productivity, and can be accessed at: http://www .businessgrouphealth.org/services/4_Part_Guide.pdf.

Partnership for Prevention, "Leading by Example." Washington, DC. This 2005 issue paper discusses the importance of employer investment in health through prevention and disease management. Although savings per dollar invested in worksite health promotion programs are difficult to quantify, the authors report that each dollar invested in worksite health programs brought savings of $3.48 in reduced health care costs and $5.82 in lower absenteeism costs. Information about *Partnership for Prevention* can be accessed at www.prevent.org.

CHAPTER 7

Early Attempts at Rationing in the United States

A New Machine for Kidney Disease

Hull, Alan R. "The Legislative and Regulatory Process in the End-Stage Renal Disease (ESRD) Program, 1973–1997." "Seminars in Nephrology" 17(3) (1997): 160–169. This article traces the development of health policy regarding paying for the treatment of kidney disease with dialysis in the U.S. and its adoption as a condition under Medicare in 1972. Estimates of the cost of the program as well as the numbers of people eligible for the service were grossly underestimated, and by the 1990s, the program utilized five percent of Medicare funds for less than one-half of one percent of

Medicare's population. See also Greer, Joel, Health Care Financing Review, Summer 2003: http://www.cms.hhs.gov/apps/review/03summer/default.asp, which gives an overview of the current End Stage Renal Disease Program under Medicare, including cost estimates and percent of population served.

The Oregon Rationing Experiment

Oberlander, John, Theodore Marmor, and Lawrence Jacobs. "Rationing Medical Care: Rhetoric and Reality in the Oregon Health Plan." CMAJ 164(11) (2001): 1583–1587. The authors describe the Oregon Health Plan (OHP) and believe that the rationing experiment failed. They cite five main conclusions about the OHP: (1) there was no widespread rationing of services, mainly because of the difficulty of taking previously provided services off the list; (2) physicians "gamed" the allocation rules under the OHP and continued to provide previously covered services; (3) there was little to no cost savings as a result of the OHP; (4) controversies among various constituencies as well as the federal government about which services would be covered forced inclusion of services that originally were not recommended, which eroded the original philosophy that only services meeting a cost-effectiveness threshold would be included; and (5) despite the OHP's attention as a U.S. policy innovation, no other state has tried the Oregon model, which may signal that a true rationing model based on a prioritized ranking is currently unacceptable in the U.S.

Bodenheimer, Thomas. "The Oregon Health Plan—Lessons for the Nation, Part I." New England Journal of Medicine 337(9) (1997): 651–655. This article gives a brief history of the development of the Oregon Health Plan and its list of health services, and discusses the change required in the structure of the Medicaid program in Oregon. Although the program faced many implementation challenges, the author believes that the Oregon Health Plan achieved its primary goal of reducing the number of uninsured citizens in the state. Between 1991 and 1995 the number of uninsured Oregonians dropped by about fifteen percent, even as the rate was rising nationally.

Gostin, Lawrence O. "The Americans with Disabilities Act and the U.S. Health System." Health Affairs (Fall 1992): 248–257. Gostin begins by defining "disabled" and speaks about the initial effect of the Americans with Disabilities Act with regard to rationing within the Oregon Health Plan.

Rationing and Insurance Coverage

Steinberg Earl P., Sean Tunis, and David Shapiro. "Insurance Coverage for Experimental Technologies." Health Affairs 14(4) (1995): 144–158. This article discusses the importance of weighing all the factors of a new technology (effectiveness and risks as defined by well-designed research studies, the overall costs of widespread use of the new technology, avoiding harm to patients, and return on investment) when developing payment policies for a new treatment or device. The authors point out that Medicare has paid for some "experimental" technologies for years, and defends the policy based on the need to "study" the safety and effectiveness of new treatments.

Lee, Kerry L., Robert M. Califf, John Simes, Frans Van de Werf, Eric J. Topol. "Holding GUSTO Up to the Light." Annals of Internal Medicine 120(10) (1994): 876–881. The Global Utilization of Streptokinase and Tissue Plasminogen Activator for Occluded Coronary Arteries (GUSTO) trial was a clinical trial looking at therapies for heart attacks. The research showed a decrease in mortality for certain patients treated with Tissue Plasminogen Activator, but the authors note that questions have been raised about whether the high cost of the new treatment ($1,000 higher than older therapy) justified its use in general clinical practice since there was only a one-percent benefit in survival.

Morrisey, Michael A. et al. "Small Employers and the Health Insurance Market." Health Affairs (Winter 1994): 149–160. This article talks about the effect of preexisting conditions on the decision of small employers to offer health insurance. Based on a survey of the benefits offered by small businesses, the authors report that one-third of employers were afraid to change insurance companies because of preexisting condition clauses. The study also found that the preexisting condition exclusions were present in both large and small employers, with similar restrictions that included wait times for certain services of one year or less.

Hennessy, Kevin D. and Howard H. Goldman. "Full Parity: Steps toward Treatment Equity for Mental and Addictive Disorders." Health Affairs 20(4) (2001): 58–67. This article discusses the 1996 Mental Health Parity Act and the effect it has had on states' insurance coverage. It details how certain states developed policies to cover only "biological" mental health disorders (e.g., schizophrenia and bipolar disorder), and excluding conditions such as substance abuse.

Barry, Colleen L., Jon R. Gabel, Richard G. Frank, Samantha Hawkins, Heidi H. Whitmore, and Jeremy D. Pickreign. "Design of Mental Health Benefits: Still Unequal After All These Years." Health Affairs 22(5) (2003): 127–137. This article examines recent trends in the design and organization of coverage for mental health care as reported through a national employer survey. The authors report that legislation and changes in the delivery of mental health services have changed how mental health insurance is bought and sold, and that access has increased, but that mental health coverage is still not offered at a level equivalent to coverage for other medical conditions. In addition, cost-sharing by the patient is higher for mental health services, creating a rationing mechanism that leads to barriers to care.

Mechanic, David and Scott Bilder. "Treatment of People with Mental Illness: A Decade-Long Perspective." Health Affairs 23(4) (2004): 84–95. The authors discuss improvements in access to mental health services over the last decade, particularly for those with the most serious conditions. Despite advances, there are more seriously mentally ill persons who are uninsured, thus limiting their access to appropriate mental health services. The authors highlight the urgent need for a greater focus on measurement of health outcomes for those with mental illness.

Bergthold, Linda A. "Medical Necessity: Do We Need It?" Health Affairs 14(4) (1995): 180–190. The term "medical necessity" has been used for more than thirty years to define what is, and is not, covered by health insurance. During the 1990s, insurance companies used the term to control the use of medical care, particularly in the area of new or experimental therapies. This article gives a brief history of the term, shows how new treatments have challenged the definition of "medically necessary," and suggests new language with clear criteria for coverage and a fair process for resolving disputes.

Garber, Alan M. "Evidence-Based Coverage Policy." Health Affairs 20(5) (2001): 62–82. This article talks about how insurance coverage is usually determined on the basis of "effectiveness, reasonableness, and necessity." Garber explains that coverage decisions are generally tied to determinations that care be "medically necessary" and based on "evidence-based" medicine, both of which depend upon the systematic review regarding the effectiveness of specific treatments. Evidence-based coverage decisions are inconsistent in part because of the differences in deciding the evidence necessary to determine both effectiveness and cost-effectiveness of medical care. Nevertheless, the author concludes that evidence evaluation will continue to evolve and be used to address both the need for cost control and the need for quality assurance in the U.S. health care system.

The Rest of the World Also Rations

Heinzl, Mark and Christopher J. Chipello. "Shock Treatment for Canadian Health Care." Wall Street Journal, June 13, 2005, page B3. This article reports on the 2005 Canadian Supreme Court ruling that Quebec's prohibition on private insurance for services covered by the public system violates the province's bill of rights that promises access to needed medical care. The case stemmed from a lawsuit alleging that a year-long wait for a hip replacement failed to meet the statutory standard of timely access to medical care.

Mechanic, David. "Muddling Through Elegantly: Finding the Proper Balance in Rationing." Health Affairs 16(5) (1997): 83–91. This article gives an overview of rationing in the U.S. and defines the difference between "implicit" rationing (elective decisions based on specific situations) and "explicit" rationing (with specific rules that everyone knows). The U.S. health system utilizes implicit rationing models; other developed countries rely on more explicit rationing models to distribute and pay for medical services. The author argues in favor of implicit over explicit rationing because of its flexibility in taking into account patient preferences and values, and because it allows discretion in determining what medical care should be provided to whom. In addition, implicit rationing may align better with the U.S. values of pluralism and rescue, even if it leads to preferential treatment for some. However, the author also acknowledges that a significant danger of implicit rationing is the tendency to promote non-standardized or inequitable care, and that checks and balances will be required to ensure efficiency, quality, and fairness.

CHAPTER 8

How Are Medical Decisions Made?

"Rating the Strength of Scientific Research Findings." Agency for Healthcare Research and Quality. No. 02-PO22 (2002). This fact sheet provides and explains different methods of analyzing medical evidence.

"Cardiac Arrhythmia Suppression Trial (CAST)." National Heart, Lung and Blood Institute (1998). http://www.clinicaltrials.gov. This article summarizes the randomized, double-blind "CAST" study, which tested four

drugs and a placebo to evaluate which drug reduced the chance of premature heartbeats. In 1987, the study began with 4,400 patients who had had a heart attack. The study was eventually stopped in 1991 when it was found, contrary to accepted opinion and popular belief, that all three drugs actually increased mortality and sudden cardiac death.

Priori Sylvia G., Werner Klein, Jean-Pierre Bassand. "Medical Practice Guidelines: Separating science from economics." European Heart Journal 24 (2003): 1962–1964. This article from the European Society of Cardiology discusses the history and importance of medical practice guidelines in cardiovascular care and in quality measurement. The authors discuss the risks of practicing medicine by what "seems logical" and by continuing certain practices based on assumptions. They cite the CAST trial as an example of how carefully conducted clinical research may uncover outcomes that were not predicted.

"High Blood Pressure Drug Less Effective than Diuretic." Medical College of Wisconsin. March 11, 2000. http://healthlink.mcw.edu/article/ 952653089. The ALLHAT (Antihypertenive and Lipid Lowering Treatment to Prevent Heart Attack) studied the effect of three blood-pressure-lowering drugs on over 42,000 patients. The study found that one of the new drugs wasn't as effective and was more costly than traditional diuretic medications. As a result of the study, recommendations on how to treat high blood pressure (for some patients) changed and cautioned physicians about introducing new types of treatment into clinical care without evaluating the effectiveness alongside older, less expensive drugs with documented benefits.

Hrobjartsson, Asbjorn and Peter Gotzshe. "Is the Placebo Powerless?" New England Journal of Medicine 344(12) (2001): 1594–1601. Placebo treatments have been reported to help patients with many conditions, and this article examines the quality of the evidence supporting the use of placebos in patient care. The researchers found that placebos had little or no significant clinical effects, except for the treatment of pain, where there may be a small benefit. The authors suggest that placebos have a place in blinded randomized clinical trials because they may help eliminate biases.

Wennberg, John E. et al. "Use of Medicare Claims Data to Monitor Provider-Specific Performance among Patients with Severe Chronic Illness." Health Affairs (2004): VAR5-18. This paper documents that the seven hospitals leading U.S. News and World Report's 2001 rankings for care of the elderly had quite different levels of care (high intensity versus low intensity) with those receiving the highest intensity of care (as measured by longer in-hospital stays and higher number of days in the intensive care unit during the last six months of life) had no better and often worse outcomes. They reference an additional study, in which patients with chronic conditions received twice as much hospital-based care over a three-year period in Boston compared with New Haven (see E. S. Fisher et al, "Hospital Readmission Rates for Cohorts of Medicare Beneficiaries in Boston and New Haven," *New England Journal of Medicine* 331(15) (2004): 989–995; and E. S. Fisher et al, "The Implications of Regional Variations in Medicare Spending, Parts 1 and 2," *Annals of Internal Medicine* Vol. 138(4) (2003): 273–298).

Practice Guidelines and Evidence-Based Medicine

Eddy, David M. "Evidence-Based Medicine: A Unified Approach." Health Affairs 24(1) (2005): 9–1. This article presents an approach to understanding the issues involving the differences between treating individual patients and developing guidelines for populations. The author believes that using evidence-based guidelines in the treatment of individual patients with "evidence-based medicine" is important because it will provide a mechanism to tailor guidelines to individual cases. The author references the landmark study that reported that only fifteen percent of medical practices were based on solid clinical trials.

Carey, J. "Medical Guesswork." BusinessWeek, May 29, 2006, 73–79. Drawing on the work of David Eddy and other researchers, this article discusses the lack of evidence for the use of many widely used treatments and procedures in medicine today. Although there has been progress in recent years, only fifteen percent of what doctors routinely do is backed by hard evidence, and only twenty to twenty-five percent of medicine is proven effective. This leads to wasted resources, inappropriate care, and a continuation of variation in how medicine is practiced. The experts quoted within the article call for a greater use of evidence-based medicine based on the randomized clinical trial, when possible, and when not, relying on computer simulations and increased patient education to encourage appropriate, scientifically based, patient-centered care.

Timmermans, Stephan and Aaron Mauck. "The Promises and Pitfalls of Evidence-Based Medicine." Health Affairs (2005): 18–27. This article begins by explaining evidence-based medicine (EBM) and how practice guidelines are created. Since more than 1,000 guidelines are produced each year, many for the same disease, it is difficult to assess which ones are more appropriate and effective. In fact, the authors state that there are so many guidelines now there is a need to create guidelines for the guidelines. Double-blind, randomized controlled trials are the "gold standard" for determining whether the evidence a study produces is sound. The article examines opposing views about EBM and practice guidelines. Opponents claim that EBM is "cookbook medicine." Some see EBM as the "deprofessionalization" of medicine. The article states that only fifty percent of physicians adhere to the guidelines.

Evidence-Based Medicine Working Group. "Evidence-Based Medicine." 268(17) (1992): 2420–2425. This paper traces the history the shift away from expert and experience-related models toward evidence-based medicine and asserts that blind comparison trials are the "gold standard" and that only randomized experiments will provide useful information.

Bergman, David A. "Evidence-Based Guidelines and Critical Pathways for Quality Improvement." Pediatrics 103(1) (1999): 225–232. This article discusses the role of EBM and practice guidelines as generated by the Academy of Pediatrics for use in children. It describes the different types of trials that one can do to determine the strength of evidence, from randomized controlled variables (the best method) to expert opinions (the worst method). Despite knowing that the best evidence comes from randomized controlled trials, only eleven percent of pediatric guidelines are generated from that source, with the majority coming from expert opinion (seventy-two percent). The authors conclude by saying that while practice guidelines are helpful tools to standardize medical care and base treatment on evidence, they do not yet provide a complete model for improving health since they are still not yet based upon appropriate trials.

Shekelle, Paul G. et al. "Validity of the Agency for Health Care Research an Quality Clinical Practice Guidelines." JAMA 286(12) (2001): 1461–1467. In this study, the authors state that practice guidelines need to be up to date to be useful to clinicians, then they examined a sample of seventeen guidelines published by the federal Agency for Healthcare Research and Quality (AHRQ) that were still in circulation. The authors found that the majority of the seventeen guidelines needed minor or major revisions and updating, and recommended that guidelines should be reassessed every three years. At the time of the article, the National Guidelines Clearing House at AHRQ held more than 1,000 guidelines. For more information about Clinical Practice

Guidelines (CPGs), go to: http://www.guideline.gov/browse/guideline_index .aspx. This website, sponsored by the federal government Agency for Health Care Research and Quality provides a complete list of guideline summaries available through the National Guideline Clearinghouse website. The listing of over 1,700 guidelines is organized alphabetically, by organization name.

Translating Evidence into Medical Practice

Fuchs, Victor R. "More Variation in Use of Care, More Flat-of-the-Curve Medicine." Health Affairs (Web Exclusive October 2, 2004): VAR104-107. This article discusses the variation in use of health care, and the resulting variation in cost and quality. The author suggests that although there is good reason to continue efforts to reduce variation in medical care and to pursue quality improvement through measuring outcomes, he doubts than any large-scale change will come until there is major reform of the health care financing system and the use of sufficient incentives for physicians and hospitals to do less and to change the way medical care is delivered.

Eagle, Kim et al. "Closing The Gap Between Science And Practice: The Need For Professional Leadership." Health Affairs (2003): 196–201. This article discusses the ongoing challenges in aligning clinical science and clinical practice. Although the insurance industry uses guidelines for financial and quality management, professional medical societies (who most often produce guidelines) have not taken a leadership role in making sure those guidelines are actually practiced. The authors cite the experience of an American College of Cardiology–sponsored project as a model to examine how guidelines can be integrated into patient care. The authors believe that specialty societies should work with others in the quality improvement industry (for example, software companies) to encourage the integration of clinical guidelines into medical practice.

Clancy, Carolyn M. and Kelly Cronin. "Evidence-Based Decision Making: Global Evidence, Local Decisions." Health Affairs 24(1) (2005): 151–162. The authors cite the problems with variation in treatment patterns in the current medical care system and say that this variation is wasteful. The authors recommend developing information systems with electronic medical records available where care is delivered, and that have the capacity to distribute health information.

Audet, Anne-Marie J., Michelle M. Dotyk, Jamil Shamasdin, and Stephen C. Schoenbaum. "Measure, Learn, and Improve: Physicians' Involvement in

Quality Improvement." *Health Affairs* 24(3) (2005): 843–853. This article summarizes a national survey assessing whether physicians use their own results to assess their performance. The results indicate that most physicians do not use such data or participate in quality improvement activities, although physicians in larger and salaried groups are more likely to use quality improvement methods.

Shojania, Kaveh G., and Jeremy M. Grimshaw. "*Evidence-based Quality Improvement: The State of the Science.*" *Health Affairs* 24(1) (2005): 138–150. Routine medical practice fails to incorporate evidence in a timely and reliable fashion, and quality improvement activities can help bridge the gaps between research and clinical care.

Perry, Seymour and Eric S. Marx. "*Practice Guidelines: Roles of Economics and Physicians.*" *Health Affairs* (1994): 141–145. The authors state that evidence-based medicine and practice guidelines should incorporate economics into their results to increase efficiency, which in turn will reduce health care costs. The authors cite the earlier RAND study that says that one-fourth to one-third of U.S. health care dollars buy care that has "marginal benefit."

CHAPTER 9

Toward a Definition of Quality

Davis, Karen et al. "*A 2020 Vision of Patient-Centered Primary Care.*" *Journal General Internal Medicine* 20(10) (2005): 953–957. The authors cite the results of the Commonwealth Fund's National Survey of Physicians and Quality of Care, where only one-fourth of primary care physicians currently consider "patient-centeredness" (i.e., inclusion of the patient's wishes) in their practices. They call for new payment structures that reward patient-centered performance.

U.S. Department of Health and Human Services. "*HHS Issues Report on Community Health in Rural, Urban Areas.*" September 10, 2001. *http://www.hhs.gov/news/press/2001press*. This report highlights community health in rural and urban areas, and indicates that the highest death rates for children and young adults were in the most rural counties. Residents of rural areas had the highest death rates for unintentional injuries generally and for motor-vehicle injuries specifically. Teenagers and adults in rural counties were the most likely to smoke, had the fewest visits for dental care, and, similar to those who live in inner cities, had low levels of insurance.

"Crossing the Quality Chasm: A New Health System for the 21st Century." Institute of Medicine (March 2001). http://www.iom.edu. This report sets goals to improve the quality of U.S. health care. These six goals include delivering safe, effective, patient-centered, timely, efficient, and equitable care. See endnotes 2 and 3 in Chapter 5 for a complete discussion of this reference and the accompanying article regarding the IOM report, *Berwick, Donald M. "A User's Manual for the IOM's 'Quality Chasm' Report." Health Affairs 21(3) (2002): 80–90.*

"To Err is Human: Building a Safer Health System." Institute of Medicine, November 1999. http://www.iom.edu. This report cited the now famous statistic that 44,000-98,000 people die as a result of preventable medical errors each year. In addition, the IOM estimates that preventable medical errors cost $17–$29 billion a year. The report offers suggestions about how to decrease preventable medical errors. Some providers feel that threat of a lawsuit stands in the way of decreasing medical errors because open discussion of errors or potential errors does not occur. The Institute of Medicine calls for mandatory and voluntary reporting systems for errors as well as a minimum standard of performance measurement for medical licensure. For popular editorials discussing medical errors and numbers of deaths per day and per hospital, see: Newt Gringrich, "High-Tech Cure for Medical Mistakes," Washington Post, August 2, 2000, page A31; and Donald M. Berwick, "Invisible Injuries," Washington Post, July 29, 2003, page A17.

The Patient's Guide to Quality

Berwick D., Lucian Leape. "Reducing Errors in Medicine." Quality in Health Care 8 (1999): 145–146. This editorial reports that serious medication errors occur in 6.7 out of every 100 patients hospitalized, with injuries from medical care itself occurring in 3.7 percent of hospital admissions, over half of which were preventable and 13.6 percent of which led to death. The authors state that these rates are no lower in other developed countries, and call for international efforts to improve patient safety through the development of error-reporting systems, safe use of medical equipment and devices, team training in patient care, and the use of innovative technologies.

National Coalition on Health Care, "Facts on the Quality of Health Care." http://www.nchc.org/facts/quality.shtml. This fact sheet, drawn from the health care quality academic and professional literature, compiles statistics regarding health care quality problems, medical errors that lead to patient death and injuries, including hospital-acquired infections, and the recommendations for system improvements to improve health care quality in the United States.

Steinbrook, Robert M.D. "Searching for the Right Search—Researching the Medical Literature." New England Journal of Medicine 354(1) (2006). Eight out of ten Internet users research health advice on the Internet using a variety of academic, public, and private sources. Areas of interest in the Internet searches include diet, fitness, drugs, health insurance, experimental treatments, and particular doctors and hospitals.

Kizer, Kenneth. "The Volume-Outcome Conundrum." New England Journal of Medicine, 349(22) (2003): 2159–2161. This article discusses the evidence that complex treatments or high-risk surgical procedures have lower death rates and better outcomes if care is provided in hospitals that have higher volumes of those treatments. The author suggests that the available evidence supports the relationship of higher volume to better outcomes, particularly when selecting physicians.

Wicks, Elliot and Jack A. Meyer. "Making Report Cards Work." Health Affairs 18(2) (1999): 152–155. This report discusses the effectiveness of report cards on health plans and providers' performance and consumers' preferences about the content of the report cards. Participants focused more on customer service rather than the quality of the medical care received. The authors give examples of companies that use report cards and provide financial incentives/disincentives for choosing quality health plans. The authors state that consumer willingness to read quality reports, understandability and accuracy of the reports, as well as incentives to the consumer for reading the data are necessary for report cards to be effective in a competitive health care market.

Bates, David W. and Atul A. Gawande. "The Impact of the Internet on Quality Measurement." Health Affairs 19(8) (2000): 104–114. This article talks about current quality measurement programs and efforts. It also discusses the pros and cons of using report cards and cautions the reader to balance the advantages of accessibility to reports and measures of health outcomes with the limitations of the data. It is important to see if the data are current as more Americans turn to the Internet to find quality information. There are more than 17,000 health-related websites that report quality data on health care professionals and organizations, and some, like HealthGrades.com, have specific information regarding individual doctors. The authors suggest developing and using standards for all Internet information so that information is less biased or incorrect, and so that it can be compared across sites.

Studdert, David M. et al. "Defensive Medicine among High-Risk Specialist Physicians in a Volatile Malpractice Environment." JAMA 293(21) (2005): 2609–2617. This study, based on a survey of physicians, looked at whether and how often physicians practiced defensive medicine because of the threat of malpractice liability, particularly among those practitioners in high-liability specialties such as obstetrics and surgery. The authors found that physicians who practiced in high-risk specialties in states with high malpractice insurance nearly always (ninety-three percent) practiced defensive medicine or avoided patients who had complex medical problems or who were perceived as likely to sue.

Grades, Rankings, and Report Cards

Green, Jesse and Neil Wintfeld. "Report Cards on Cardiac Surgeons— Assessing New York State's Approach." New England Journal of Medicine 332 (1995): 1229–1233. This article discusses the emergence of hospital and individual physician "report cards" ranking patient outcomes for various clinical treatments, and discusses the use of cardiac surgery "mortality" reports in New York State. New York and Pennsylvania were the first states to offer the controversial practice of publishing physician-specific mortality rates among patients who undergo heart surgery. The authors suggest caution in the use of such report cards because accurate comparison of health outcomes data remains challenging due to the problems of risk-adjustment techniques to compensate for the care of sicker patients and because of the problems of missing data. The authors conclude that in order to ensure that report cards provide fair comparisons among physicians and provide standardized information for patients, the methods and data used in report cards should be independently evaluated on a regular basis.

"Physician Quality Report." Healthgrades.com. This is a sample of the information that one can obtain from Healthgrades.com. *Healthgrades* provides information about specific physicians. It is an easy-to-use website that allows a search for physicians by state, city, and name. For a fee, the website will provide professional background, board certification, government disciplinary actions, a comparison of the physicians to national statistics, patient satisfaction survey, and physician characteristics.

"The "Best Doctors in America" list (found at http://medicalcenter.osu .edu/patientcare/findadoctor/best/) is considered to be one of the more prestigious and credible lists of outstanding physicians available to consumers for selecting a doctor. The survey, developed using evaluations by physicians and updated every two years, includes physicians in primary care and specialty areas, such as cardiology, surgery, and pediatrics.

Vara, Vauhini. *"Sites Offering Data, Reviews of Doctors." Wall Street Journal Online, www.wsj.com, November 23, 2005.* This article lists websites that offer information on or reviews of doctors. Sites include: AMA's *DoctorFinder;* Administrators in Medicine *DocFinder;* Federation of State Medical Boards Physician Data Center; *HealthGrades.com; RateMDs.com; DoctorOogle.com; and DrScore.com.* Some of the websites offer information free of charge, and others charge a fee for information about specific physician reviews.

NCQA Overview. http://www.ncqa.org. The National Commission on Quality Assurance (NCQA), like the JCAHO, is an accreditation organization that measures quality of care in managed care organizations, but also has programs that target hospital and individual providers. The NCQA developed the Health Plan-Employer Data Information Set (HEDIS), which contains over sixty different performance measures in the areas of preventive services (for example, immunizations, screenings, and chronic care management), patient safety, confidentiality, consumer protection, access, service, and continued quality improvement. HEDIS measures are used by more than ninety percent of health maintenance organizations (HMOs) as a way to measure their performance and as a way to provide "apples to apples" comparisons between HMOs, which then should permit consumers to able to choose higher performing health plans.

Schneider, Eric C. et al. *"National Quality Monitoring of Medicare Health Plans." Medical Care 39(12): 1313–1325.* Starting in 1997, the federal government has required HMOs that participate in Medicare to report data about their quality using the Consumer Assessment of Health Plans

Study (CAHPS) and the Health Plan-Employer Data Information Set (HEDIS). CAHPS is a national survey that focuses on health plan access and communication while HEDIS focuses on the quality of medical care and mental health care services.

"Health Grades Quality Study: Patient Safety in American Hospitals." HealthGrades Inc. 2004. This study uses hospital discharge Medicare data to determine the frequency and cost of medical errors across different hospitals. Summary of the findings include: 1.14 million total patient safety incidents (PSIs) occurred among the thirty-seven million hospitalizations (three percent) in the Medicare population from 2000 through 2002; there were variations across hospitals and regions; the errors studied accounted for $8.54 billion in excess inpatient cost to the Medicare system over three years.

Joint Commission on Accreditation of Healthcare Organizations. "Setting the Standard for Quality in Health Care." http:///www.jcaho.org . This pamphlet establishes the role of JCAHO as the oldest and largest health accreditation organization. The pamphlet explains why it is in the best interest of providers and consumers that health care organizations receive accreditation, for consumers will know that the health care they receive has passed numerous performance measurements, and accreditation for provider organizations will increase their competitiveness in the health market.

Joint Commission and Health Care Safety and Quality. "Setting the Standard." http://www.jcaho.org. In this 2005 publication, the JCAHO self reports that it is the "gold standard" in health organization accreditation. Over 15,000 providers use JCAHO's quality standards to provide care to their patients and are able to measure their performance over a period of time. This pamphlet describes many of JCAHO's initiatives, such as National Patient Safety Standards and Goals, Emergency Management Standards, and Patient Rights Standards.

National Committee for Quality Assurance. "The State of Health Care Quality 2005." Executive Summary: 6–14. This annual report from NCQA suggests providers who measure their performance continue to improve year to year. Improvements in quality of care have resulted in a decrease in the number of lives lost to medical errors. In fact, according to the annual report, since NCQA started collecting information, quality improvements such as providers prescribing beta blockers after a heart attack, cholesterol management after a heart attack, and controlling high blood pressure and diabetes' complications have saved over 50,000 lives and prevented thousands of other critical events such as second heart attacks. However, this progress is hindered by the rising cost of medical care that prompts some employers to shift away from health plans that measure quality performance to less expensive health plans that do not collect or report quality data. In fact, this year, NCQA participating plans covered 21.5 percent of Americans, down from twenty-three percent in 2004. Recognition.ncqa.org is a website created by NCQA that provides information about individual health plans.

McCormick, Danny, et al. "Relationship Between Low Quality-of-Care Scores and HMOs' Subsequent Public Disclosure of Quality-of-Care Scores." JAMA 288(12) (2002): 1484–1490. The authors found that HMO plans that score lower on quality are more likely to stop disclosing their quality data, and suggest that reporting of HMO quality data must be mandatory.

CHAPTER 10

How Do Consumers Make Decisions?

Brody, Jane E. "Just What the Doctor Ordered? Not Exactly." New York Times, May 9, 2006, www.nytimes.com. In this New York Times editorial, the author describes the problem of patients not following their doctor's prescribed medical care. The article states that at least half of all patients fail to comply with treatments their doctors prescribe—especially when it comes to medications.

California Health Care Foundation. "Consumers in Health Care: The Burden of Choice." (October 2005), 34 pages, accessed at: www.chcf.org. This report summarizes findings and best practices for organizations working to develop tools to help consumers make decisions. Key findings from the report include: (1) contrary to the popular idea that "more information is better," research shows that more information may actually make decision-making harder; (2) consumers change their minds during the decision-making process; and (3) certain individuals use their experience and others analyze new information to make decisions.

Making Decisions About Medical Care

Davis, Karen et al. "A 2020 Vision of Patient-Centered Primary Care." The Commonwealth Fund. New York, 2005. Since the Institute of Medicine report identified patient-centered care as a major aim of quality health care, it has become increasingly important to engage patients in decisions about their own medical care. This Commonwealth Fund report presents a vision for patient-centered primary care, which includes physicians as advisers and partners, and coordinating care from generalists to specialists; an information system will be required that promotes quality improvement, patient feedback, and includes publicly available information about the practice styles and health outcomes of specific health care providers. The authors note that this "vision" will require sustained effort and leadership in medicine and business in addition to changes in payment policies for primary care.

Dowd, Bryan. "Coordinated Agency versus Autonomous Consumers in Health Services Market." Health Affairs 24(6) (2005): 1501–1511. The authors of this paper argue that managed care and consumer-driven health care (CHDC) should co-exist in a fully developed health insurance marketplace. Although CDHC holds the promise that "empowered" consumers will spend their money more wisely, there will always be patients and consumers who prefer "agents" to make decisions on their behalf. This behavior is reflected in other consumer decisions such as seeking help in investments and using insurance agents. Because of this, in the author's view, consumers of health care will never be willing or able to "go it alone," either because consumers want to rely on health professionals, or because of the lack of good consumer information regarding price and quality. As such, there may be room for both managed care and CDCH models in a "consumer-driven" health insurance market.

Davis, Karen. "Consumer-Directed Health Care: Will it Improve Health System Performance?" HSR: Health Services Research 39(4), Part II (August 2004). This commentary discusses the RAND Health Insurance Experiment (HIE) study and how it applies to high-deductible health plans. The HIE demonstrated that with greater out-of-pocket costs, patients reduce the amount of care they seek, whether the care is "necessary" or not. The author suggests that having patients pay more out of pocket therefore may be especially harmful for low income and high-risk individuals, who may not seek necessary preventive care, follow-up care, or fill prescriptions. In addition, the author believes that high deductible plans will attract wealthier, healthier people who will choose less costly plans that may deliver poorer quality. This behavior could decrease the purchase of health plans that deliver high quality. In order to achieve a truly high performance health system, Davis recommends public reporting of cost and quality data on all types of health care providers (e.g., doctors, nurses, chiropractors, hospitals), investment in health information technology, development and distribution of clinical guidelines and quality standards, rewarding quality through financial "pay for performance" strategies, and investment in research to improve quality and efficiency.

Samuel, Thomas W. et al. "The Next Stage in Health Care Economy: Aligning the Interests of Patients, Providers, and Third Party Payers through Consumer-Driven Health Care Plans." The American Journal of Surgery 186 (2003): 117–124. The authors of this paper review attempt over the last twenty-five years to address the cost and accessibility of health care services. Traditionally, fee-for-service models were thought to be good for providers and patients because each benefited from more services; patients thought "more is better" and providers made more money with each service. But payers complained of increasing costs as more medical care was delivered. During managed care, payers ruled with cost reductions, while patients complained about restriction in available care and lack of choice. Most recently, in consumer-driven models, patients and payers may benefit when financial incentives result in lower out-of-pocket payments and premiums, although providers and the health of patients may suffer because of less medical care. The authors conclude by questioning whether Consumer Directed Health Care (CDHC) models will succeed in creating a more rational health system, or whether CDHC will just be the next failed attempt to control costs.

Vinn, Norman E. "The Emergence of Consumer-Driven Health Care." American Academy of Family Physicians, 2000. http://www.aafp.org. This article discusses the physician/patient relationship over the years through the various employer-sponsored health insurance models, including managed care, preferred-provider organizations (PPOs), and now Consumer Directed Health Care. As employers pass more of the costs and decisions to employees, along with information about specific providers, patients will be expected to evaluate their physicians not only for the results of their clinical care, but also for customer service, access, and value. CDHC provides new challenges and opportunities for physicians, including improving care management through patient education, but it also requires a focus on service excellence and administrative performance standards such as telephone response times, appointment wait times, and turnaround times for reporting test results.

Kristof, Nicholas D. "Take a Hike." New York Times (nytimes.com), January 31, 2006. This editorial discusses the eventual problems caused by the unhealthy diet and lifestyle of Americans, from French fry consumption (one out of five children eat French fries at least once a day) to the lack of regular exercise. The columnist suggests regulating the sale of tobacco as a drug (so that it be sold only in pharmacies), taxing junk foods (nineteen states impose taxes on particular foods like soda), promoting exercise (more bike paths) and exercise breaks at work, and expanding health education programs in schools. He ends his article by celebrating past advances in health through public health interventions, such as the use of seatbelts, greater auto safety, and anti-smoking measures, and suggests that a continued commitment to this approach today would result in tremendous future health benefits.

Wall Street Journal. "Most Americans Say Smokers Should Pay More for Insurance." WSJ Online/Harris Interactive Health-Care Poll, December 21, 2005. This health care survey conducted by Harris Interactive for the Wall Street Journal reported that a majority (sixty-three percent) of those polled think smokers and those who don't wear seatbelts should pay higher levels of insurance premiums, co-payments, or deductibles. However, while more companies are introducing different levels of insurance premiums for employees as a way to influence behaviors, the poll found tremendous opposition to this strategy. Support for the use of positive incentives such as smoking cessation programs or counseling services to encourage healthier behavior received greater support than punishment for unhealthy behaviors.

Gruber, Jonathan. "The Economics of Tobacco Regulation." Health Affairs 21(2) (2002): 146–162. Tobacco is the leading cause of preventable death in the U.S. This article examines the history of tobacco regulation and reports that since 1995 taxes on tobacco products have increased by a third, associated with a ten-percent decline in tobacco use over the same five years. Despite the fact that tobacco use saves the country money because of the premature death of smokers, tobacco regulation is justified, the authors conclude, as a public health measure, and proceeds from the sale of tobacco as well as through tobacco settlement payments might best be used in public health programs such as smoking cessation and youth smoking interventions.

Cook, Philip J. and Michael J. Moore. "The Economics of Alcohol Abuse and Alcohol Control Policies." Health Affairs 21(2) (2002): 120–133. Five percent of all deaths in the U.S. are alcohol related. This article examines alcohol regulation and the effects on the amount of alcohol consumed. Previous research suggests that increased price, in the form of an excise tax, will decrease alcohol consumption and alcohol-related problems. The authors suggest that the tax on alcohol should be higher so that it covers the cost to society of alcohol-related events.

Edgman-Levitan, Susan and Paul D. Cleary. "What Information Do Consumers Want and Need?" Health Affairs 15(4) (1996): 42–56. This article reviews information from surveys and focus group studies about how consumers define high quality care and what types of information are helpful when selecting health plans. Generally speaking, consumers are primarily interested in receiving information about the cost of care, what is covered, the quality of care, coordination of care, and access to a provider. They trust their friends' evaluations of health plans more than published "patient satisfaction" ratings. The authors conclude that physicians can help patients make good health decisions, but that will not replace the need to understand better the types of information wanted by consumers.

Lambrew, Jeanne M. "'Choice' in Health Care: What Do People Really Want?" The Commonwealth Fund Issue Brief No. 853, September 2005. This study looks at what we mean by "choice" in health care and what types of choices are important to consumers within types of health plans. The backdrop for this study is the analysis of whether proposals to expand the individual health insurance market through health savings accounts (HSAs) provide consumers with more choice. Analysis of the survey data indicated that for the patient, having a choice of health plan providers mattered most. The survey also looked at choice of a health insurance plan; those consumers in the survey who had had experience with employer-based health insurance believed that employers do a good job of selecting quality plans; two-thirds preferred that the employer select the plan rather than having the employee purchase coverage on their own. The author concludes with the caution that moving from employer-based health care to an individual system may decrease satisfaction.

University of Virginia, Consumer Health Education Institute. *Results of telephone survey as part of the Tailored Educational Approaches for Consumer Health (TEACH) Project, 2006, personal communication.* This demonstration project looks at how much health information consumers want and how they want to get the information. It included a pilot survey of more than 1,200 people conducted in the spring of 2006. Their findings suggest that approximately seventy percent would look for information from a health care professional, and eighty-eight percent stated that they trusted information from a health care professional. Three out of four respondents (seventy-four percent) replied that they would likely go to their health care professional in the future for medical information.

Consumer-Directed Health Care and High Deductible Plans

Robinson, James C. *"Health Savings Accounts—The Ownership Society in Health Care." New England Journal of Medicine 353(12) (2005): 1199–1202.* This perspective explains how health savings accounts (HSAs) are structured, and the role they play in the current health care debate surrounding the role of the individual to take "ownership" of his or her health. This is in contrast to the traditional model of health insurance that spreads risk across a large number of people and therefore is able to provide payment for sicker individuals. Through HSAs, individuals save up for their own medical care needs; HSAs give consumers/patients greater control over their medical care decisions. The author admits that this process may work well for people who can understand and manage health care decisions, but may not work so well for people who do not understand or are not comfortable making these types of medical decisions. Although consumer-driven products like HSAs may decrease the overuse of health services, the author suggests that it may also cause patients to avoid necessary medical care such as preventive care, follow-up visits to the physician, and filling prescriptions for medication. In his view, HSAs, as part of an "ownership society" philosophy, weakens society's sense of collective responsibility as it emphasizes the importance of individual effort.

Rosenthal, Meredith and Charleen Hsuan, and Arnold Milstein. *"A Report Card on the Freshman Class of Consumer-Directed Health Plans." Health Affairs 24(6) (2004): 1592–1600.* This article examines consumer-directed health plans that offer spending accounts in order to evaluate whether they were likely to reduce health care spending and improve the value of spending for health benefits. The authors found major weaknesses in these types of plans: they do not provide adequate consumer information in order to make good decisions, there are not appropriate financial incentives such as maximum benefit levels to control spending after the deductible is met, and they lack safeguards to encourage the use of preventive services, particularly for low-income populations.

McNeill, Dwight. "Do Consumer-Directed Health Benefits Favor the Young and Healthy?" Health Affairs 23(1) (2004): 186–193. The study analyzes consumers' out-of-pocket payments for health insurance premiums and medical care and found that consumer-directed health plans (CDHPs) favor the young and healthy, who are potential "winners" with CDHPs, and the moderately sick are the "losers," partly because when asked to use their own money for medical services, people use less of both appropriate and inappropriate services, and therefore the moderately sick will use less necessary care. A possible fix to these problems in CDHPs lies in limiting the out-of-pocket payments as a percentage of income (for example, five percent), as is done in most European countries.

Brewer, Benjamin. "A Family Doctor Adapts to Health Savings Accounts." The Doctor's Office, Wall Street Journal Online (www.wsj.com), January 24, 2006. This Wall Street Journal column by a family doctor highlights his experience with patients who have converted to a health savings account. Dr. Brewer praises the use of such health savings accounts for his patients who are relatively healthy or who don't have access to more comprehensive employer-sponsored health insurance, but he says that there can be problems when patients question the need for care in order to save money. In one example, the author relates the experience of convincing a mother that her child with pneumonia needed a chest x-ray and blood work.

Davis, K., M. Doty, and A Ho. "How High Is Too High? Implications of High Deductible Health Plans," Pub. No 816 (New York: Commonwealth Fund, 2005). This study examines high-deductible health plans (HDHP) compared with traditional health insurance, and reports that although HDHPs may increase access to affordable health insurance, they do not necessarily reduce financial burden in those with poor health or those with low income. The study finds the following information about people who have high-deductible health insurance: thirty-eight percent of adults did not fill a prescription, did not get specialist care, did not follow up on care, or did not seek necessary care; fifty-four percent of adults with deductibles of over $1,000 had difficulty paying medical bills or had debt due to bills; and low-income individuals and families at twice the federal poverty level (approximately $40,000 for a family of four) could spend twenty-six percent of their income before reaching the ceiling on out-of-pocket expenses. The authors suggest that one change that insurers could make to improve high-deductible plans is paying for preventive and primary care services separately from the plan's deductible—thus not discouraging the use of preventive or primary care services.

Fuhrmans, Vanessa. "More Employers Try Limited Health Plans." Wall Street Journal Online (www.wsj.com), January 17, 2006. This article reports on the growing use of low-cost "mini-medical" or "limited-benefit" plans, traditionally used as bridge health coverage plans for people between jobs, but now used more extensively as employers struggle with the rising cost of health insurance. To date, over one million people have such plans, which typically cover four to ten doctor visits a year, a certain amount of prescription drugs, and some lab tests. Critics say that consumers don't always understand the limitations of these policies, including the lack of coverage for hospital care or annual maximum payment by the plan. These types of plans promote confusion, particularly among consumers purchasing them without the guidance of an employer's human resource department, and may open the door to brokers who may misrepresent the benefits.

CHAPTER II

Can You See Your Doctor?

Cooper, Richard, et al. "Economic and Demographic Trends Signal an Impending Physician Shortage." Health Affairs 21(1) (2002): 140–154. The author suggests in this article, bucking the "conventional wisdom" of the time in 2002, that the U.S. was about to experience a shortage of physicians. Using a new model for workforce planning based on economic expansion, population growth, physicians' work effort, and the services provided by nonphysician clinicians (such as nurses), the author predicts that the U.S. would have to create twenty-five new medical schools over the next ten years in order to meet the growing demand for physician services.

Snyderman, Ralph et al. "Gauging Supply and Demand: The Challenging Quest to Predict the Future Physician Workforce." Health Affairs 21(1) (2002): 167–168. The authors review previous workforce planning studies of the early 1990s where physician future supply needs were projected based upon health maintenance organization (HMO) staffing patterns—a model that used many fewer specialists and fewer physicians overall. These early studies predicted a surplus of 150,000 physicians, and virtually all major physician organizations responded by stating that the country was on the verge of a serious oversupply of physicians. Since then, the authors note that other experts have come forward with predictions that the U.S. will face a grave undersupply of physicians in the next twenty years, a trend they say is more likely.

Blumenthal, David. "New Steam from an Old Cauldron—The Physician Supply Debate." New England Journal of Medicine 350(17) (2004): 1780–1787. This article gives a history of the physician supply in the U.S. beginning back in the early part of the twentieth century, and traces the ups and downs in American workforce planning. From the early 1980s to the mid-1990s professional organizations measuring future physician supply needs forecasted a surplus, but, in the late 1990s, there was a shift toward the belief that the U.S. was facing a physician shortage, particularly for specialists. These beliefs were supported by surveys from New York and California that reported specialists having 1.3 times as many job offers as generalists. The author concludes that there are many variables in predicting physician workforce needs as well as difficulties increasing the supply of physicians, including public investment in medical training and the inability of many medical schools to appreciably increase their numbers of medical students.

Girion, Lisa. "Needs of Patients Outpace Doctors." Los Angeles Times, June 4, 2006, accessed at www.latimes.com. This article describes the impending physician shortage in California and the U.S., and suggests that the shortage will create access, quality, and cost problems throughout the health system. Some of the signs of the growing need for more physicians include: twelve states report current or expected shortages, particularly in cardiology, radiology, and surgical subspecialties; the aging of the physician workforce and the increased rate of physician retirements (22,000 retirements a year by 2020 compared with 9,000 in 2000); the entrance of women into the profession along with a greater desire by younger physicians—both male and female—to work fewer hours, suggesting a ten-percent decrease in productivity; the longer wait times for appointments to see physicians; and the increased demand for procedures like cataract surgery from an aging population. Although there is a recommendation for medical schools to increase their enrollment by thirty percent, the author reports that the president of the Association of American Medical Colleges (AAMC) states that even if schools could increase capacity by thirty percent, the ratio of physicians to patients would begin to decline by 2025.

American Association of Medical Colleges. "The Supply of Physician Services in OECD Countries. "OECD, Steven Simoens & Jeremy Hurst. Health Working Papers." Prepared by AAMC Center for Workforce Studies, January 2006. This report cites that the per-capita number of physicians in the U.S. is lower than most developed countries and that the U.S. ranks thirteenth among the twenty OECD countries.

Trends in Physician Supply and Demand: Supply

Council on Graduate Medical Education, 16th Annual Report, "Physician Workforce Policy Guidelines for the United States 2000–2020." U.S. Department of Health and Human Services, Health Resources and Services Administration, January 2005. This publication reports on many issues surrounding physician workforce in the U.S., including the supply and geographic distribution of physicians in the U.S.; current and future shortages or excesses of physicians in medical and surgical specialties and subspecialties; issues relating to international medical school graduates; appropriate federal policies with respect to physician supply and distribution; appropriate roles for hospitals, schools of "Allopathic Medicine" (leading to the MD degree) and schools of "Osteopathic Medicine" (leading to the DO degree); and needs for improvements in the monitoring of the physician workforce. The recommendations of the report include: (1) increase the number of physicians entering residency training; (2) increase total enrollment in U.S. medical schools by fifteen percent; (3) increase the number of residency positions eligible for funding from Medicare to parallel the increase in U.S. medical school graduates; (4) develop systems to track the supply, demand, need, and distribution of physicians; (5) undertake specialty-specific studies to better understand the physician workforce needs; (6) promote efforts to increase the productivity of physicians (particularly advances in information technology); and (7) expand programs that address geographic

distribution of physicians, improved access to care for underserved populations and communities, appropriate distribution of physicians in various
specialties, and the promotion of workforce diversity.

U.S. Department of Health and Human Services, Health Resources and
Services Administration, Bureau of Health Professionals. "Shortage Designation," accessed January 30, 2006, at http://bhpr.hrsa.gov/shortage/. The
Health Professional Shortage Areas (HPSA) designation means that there
are shortages of primary, dental, and mental health care professionals in either urban or rural areas. An area is defined as a HPSA if the physician to
patient ratio is 1:3500. Twenty percent of the U.S. population lives in a
health professional shortage area.

Goodman, David C. "Twenty-Year Trends in Regional Variations in the
U.S. Physician Workforce." Health Affairs (Web Exclusive October 7, 2004):
VAR90-97. Large differences in the regional supply of physicians make
methods of determining the "right" workforce rate difficult. This study indicates that most physicians locate in regions with an already large supply,
and that there is as much as a 300-percent variation across regions. Because
of these differences, the author suggests that workforce planning efforts
need to factor in geographic information, or further expansions in the number of physicians may only cause high-supply regions to grow even more.

Grumbach, Kevin. "Report Offers Strategies to Remedy Chronic Shortage of Medical Care." The Center for Health Professions. May 18, 1999.
This article talks about health professional shortage areas (HPSAs) and the
reasons why physicians don't want to practice in such areas. Reasons include: low reimbursement, high-crime areas, poor facilities, isolation, and
lack of culture. The report suggests ways in which both the state and federal government can provide financial incentives to increase the number of
physicians working in HPSAs.

U.S. General Accounting Office, GAO-04-124, October 2003. "Physician
Workforce." This report describes the various federal programs to support
the training of physicians and efforts to encourage them to work in underserved geographic areas. The goals of these targeted programs include: to
improve geographic distribution of physicians; to encourage representation
of minorities in the health workforce; and to increase the overall supply of
health professionals. This article gives physician growth rates from
1991–2001 and concludes that geographic disparities in physician supply
have continued even as the national physician supply has increased steadily.

Association of American Medical Colleges. "Questions and Answers about the AAMC's New Physician Workforce Position." March 25, 2005, http://www.aamc.org/meded/cfws/start.htm. Association of American Medical Colleges. "The Physician Workforce: Position Statement." February 22, 2005. These two Association of American Medical Colleges (AAMC) reports predict that there will be a need to increase the physician supply by 2020, with estimates of need from 90,000 to 200,000 additional physicians. The AAMC says that different regions will face greater shortages than other regions, but that an overall increase in the number of physicians will be needed to address the issue of the aging of the physician population, changing expectations on the part of newly trained physicians about lifestyle, and shorter work hours. In order to meet this challenge, the AAMC calls for an increased number of residency positions funded under Medicare, continued use of graduates from foreign medical schools ("international medical graduates"), and increasing medical school enrollment by fifteen percent, or 2,500 students/year. AAMC has also recently revised this figure upward to thirty percent.

Mullan, Fitzhugh. "The Case for More U.S. Medical Students." New England Journal of Medicine 343(3) (2000): 213–217. This article focuses on the differences between the number of people attending medical school and the number of residency programs available. The number of residencies available is thirty percent greater than the number of people enrolling in medical school. This disparity implies that there are sufficient numbers of residency positions available, although there are not enough U.S. medical students to fill them. This gap is currently filled with international medical graduates (IMGs). Drawing physicians from other countries can leave the countries supplying those physicians with a shortage, but decreasing the number of IMGs while increasing the number of U.S. medical students could increase the physician shortage problems in U.S. underserved areas, since IMGs often practice in geographically underserved areas that have a hard time attracting U.S.-trained physicians.

McMahon, Graham T. "Coming to America—International Medical Graduates in the United States." New England Journal of Medicine 350(24) (2004): 2435–2437. This article describes the growth of international medical graduates (IMG) in the U.S. and states that twenty-five percent of the physicians in the U.S. are IMGs, a growth of 160 percent since 1975. The author reports that there will continue to be an ever-increasing dependence on IMGs because, although the number of physicians in the U.S. has increased at twice the rate of population growth in the past ten years, many urban and rural communities continue to have a shortage of physicians. IMGs will continue to serve an important role for those communities that have difficulty attracting U.S.-trained physicians.

Cooper, Richard A. "Weighing the Evidence for Expanding Physician Supply." Annals of Internal Medicine 141(9) (2004): 705–714. This article uses economic models and predicts a physician shortage in the near future. One of the variables examined in the study is physician work effort. The author reports that as physicians age, they work fewer hours, increasing the demand for physicians. In addition, women physicians throughout their careers work on average twenty to twenty-five percent less than men and tend to choose specialties in which time commitments are more controllable. Long-range estimates predict that by 2020, sixty percent of medical students and forty-five percent of practicing physicians will be women, suggesting that previous workforce planning models based on male work patterns would not predict future supply accurately.

Baker, Laurence. "Differences in Earnings Between Male and Female Physicians." New England Journal of Medicine 334(13) (1996): 960–964. The authors reported that female physicians work fifty hours a week for forty-six weeks and male physicians work sixty-two hours a week for forty-seven weeks.

Garson, Arthur, Stephen S. Mick, Rene Cabral-Daniels, William L. Harp. "Virginia Statewide Physician Workforce Study: Current Supply and Future Projections." January 2005. This study looked at the current supply and future projections of the physician workforce in the Commonwealth of Virginia. The study found that twenty percent of physicians planned to retire within twenty years (two percent per year); twenty-seven percent of physicians planned on reducing their patient care hours within five years, and sixty-four percent within ten years; the current patient care hours average of forty-two hours was less than historic norms.

Demand for Physicians: Why We Need More

LaMascus, Alice et al. "Bridging the Workforce Gap for Our Aging Society: How to Increase and Improve Knowledge and Training. Report of an Expert Panel." American Geriatrics Society. JAGS 53 (2005): 343–347. This article discusses the great need for geriatric medicine (those who care for the elderly) as Baby Boomers age. In the United States today, thirteen percent, or approximately thirty-five million, of our population is aged sixty-five and older. In 2011, Baby Boomers will begin turning sixty-five. Ten thousand Boomers per day will then reach this milestone over the next twenty years, and by 2030, the number of people aged sixty-five and older will have doubled to seventy-one million, representing one in five Americans. In addition, the fastest-growing segment, those aged eighty-five and older, will rise in number from four million to twenty million by 2050, and will place the greatest demand upon the medical system. Sixty percent of all Medicare beneficiaries have chronic illnesses and twenty percent of those with chronic illness have five or more chronic conditions. There are not enough physicians to care for the increasing elderly population. Reports estimate needing about 36,000 geriatric doctors, while current supply predictions will yield only 6,000. The authors state that doctors have little incentive to go into geriatrics because of low Medicare reimbursement rates. Currently, less than one percent of medical school faculty list geriatrics as their specialty.

Wolff, Jennifer L. et al. "Prevalence, Expenditures, and Complications of Multiple Chronic Conditions in the Elderly." Archives of Internal Medicine 162 (2002): 2269–2276. The study cites that forty-five percent of the general population and eighty-eight percent of the aged population have one or more chronic conditions and that the frequency of people having chronic conditions continues to increase, with estimates that 157 million Americans will have at least one chronic condition by 2020. The authors recommend better primary care and coordination of care in order to avoid hospitalizations, especially for those individuals with multiple chronic illnesses.

Ostbye, Truls et al. "Is There Time for Management of Patients with Chronic Diseases in Primary Care?" Annals of Family Medicine 3(3) (2005): 209–214. Despite the availability of national practice guidelines, many patients fail to receive recommended chronic disease care. The authors applied chronic disease guideline recommendations for ten common chronic diseases to a panel of 2,500 primary care patients and estimated the minimum physician time required to deliver high quality care for these conditions. Using these estimates, physicians would need to spend 10.6 hours a day on chronic disease management alone, for a subset of their patients, which would require more time than primary care physicians have available for patient care overall—and that is only for half their patients

Wilkinson, John M. et al. "Health Promotion in a Changing World: Preparing for the Genomics Revolution." American Journal of Health Promotion 18(2) (2003): 157–161. This article discusses the challenges after sequencing the human genome. Overall, these advances will require health professionals to create new ways to promote and recommend disease prevention. Clinicians will need to understand gene therapy and look at ways in which these types of therapy will shift the structure of medicine from diagnosis/treatment to prediction/prevention, and will also allow doctors to individualize medicine based upon a person's genetic composition. This shift will increase workload for health care practitioners.

Ojha, Rohit P. "Health Care Policy Issues as a Result of the Genetic Revolution: Implications for Public Health." American Journal of Public Health 95(3) (2005): 385–388. This article discusses how advances in genetic and molecular technology will revolutionize medicine, but also raises public policy issues in the areas of privacy, gene patenting, and education.

University of Pennsylvania, Wharton School. "Personalized Medicine and Nanotechnology: Trying to Bring Dreams to Market." Accessed March 6, 2006 at http://knowledge.wharton.upenn.edu. This article explores the many ways that the science of genetics and the use of technologies will combine and lead to medical advances in the area of "personalized medicine." Personalized medicine is the ability to formulate the precise drug or treatment that an individual patient needs and the specific techniques that are tailored to specific patients for use in a specific disease. Advances in personalized medicine include the ability to identify people who are likely to get particular diseases and to design drugs that target particular genes. This type of treatment is currently being tried in some types of cancer care.

Miller, Robert H. and Ida Sim. "Physicians' Use of Electronic Medical Records: Barriers and Solutions." Health Affairs 23(2) (2004): 116–126. This article looks at the time costs associated with electronic medical record (EMR) in physician practices. Research indicates that physicians using EMRs spent more time per patient for months or years after the EMR implementation, and the increased time costs resulted in longer workdays or fewer patients seen during the initial implementation period. Although the technology enables quality and workflow improvements over time, there are serious time and cost barriers to its adoption.

Can We Fill the Gap for More Physicians?

Cooper, Richard. "Medical Schools and their Applicants: An Analysis." Health Affairs 22(4) (2003): 71–84. Cooper predicts that the physician shortage could be as much as 200,000 doctors by 2025. One way to help the predicted shortage is to increase enrollment in medical schools, although at present there is little incentive or financial aid available for schools to do this. Historically, workforce shortages were helped by public investment in medical education. The author argues the current situation requires informing the public and legislators about the severity of the problem, requiring new public funding, and better mechanisms to attract sufficient numbers of applicants to medical schools.

Cooper, Richard A. et al. "Perceptions of Medical School Deans and State Medical Society Executives about Physician Supply." JAMA 290(22) (2003). This study surveyed medical school deans and state medical society executives to determine whether or not they perceived there was a physician shortage. Medical school deans reported that they believed there was a physician shortage, especially with regard to specialists. Of the schools surveyed, thirty percent reported that they are in the process of expanding their enrollment, thirty percent have no plans for expansion, and a few larger schools were in the process of reducing class size. Taken together, the actual and predicted future expansion was only 7.6 percent. The author notes that this is a real problem for increasing the numbers of physicians.

Bruccoleri, Rebecca. "GME Funding." 2005 American Medical Student Association. http://www.amsa.org/pdf/Medicare_GME.pdf. This brief report gives an overview of graduate medical education (GME) and GME funding. GME refers to physician specialty training that follows medical school. This primer explains the role of the Medicare program and the various funding streams that support GME, and how legislation over the past several decades has influenced the scope and quality of GME.

Croasdale, Myrle. "The 80-Hour Experience—What Happens When Residents Have to Leave." Accessed at www.ama-assn.org/amednews, July 25, 2005. This article discusses whether the Accreditation Council for Graduate Medical Education's (ACGME) 2003 regulations that required residents to limit their work hours hurt or helped educational training. These regulations state that no resident may work more than 80 hours a week. In support of the 80-hour work week, the chair of the ACGME committee cited research documenting a decrease in judgment, motor skills, and patient safety with extended work hours—longer than 80 hours.

CHAPTER 12

Problems with the Current Medical Malpractice System

Studdert, David M. et al. "Medical Malpractice." New England Journal of Medicine 350(3) (2004): 283–192. This article describes the history of the medical malpractice system and current challenges. It points out the financial power of the lawyer in this system, where approximately sixty cents of every dollar spent in medical malpractice goes toward legal fees and a small amount to administrative costs. The authors discuss the opposing roles of the patient safety and the medical malpractice movements, in which patient safety requires openness about medical mistakes and the fear of malpractice often discourages physicians from talking about and sharing medical errors. The authors discuss the various types of tort reforms including limiting access to courts by settlements, limiting claims by tightening liability rules, limiting the size of awards including ways to stop plaintiffs from being paid from multiple sources (such as insurance, that could result in double payment), and the introduction of administrative law hearings or medical courts.

Thorpe, Kenneth E. "The Medical Malpractice 'Crisis': Recent Trends and the Impact of State Tort Reforms." Health Affairs 21 (January 2004): W420-30. This article discusses how the current liability system neither improves medical care nor compensates injured patients appropriately. One study they cite found that only one malpractice claim was filed for every eight negligent medical injuries. Their analysis indicated that capping payments from malpractice awards was associated with lower premiums.

Mello, Michelle M. "Understanding Medical Malpractice Insurance: A Primer." The Robert Wood Johnson Foundation (January 2006). This report includes an overview of medical malpractice insurance, and presents sections on the history, function, and workings of the medical malpractice insurance system. The U.S. spends $6.5 billion dollars on malpractice (which translates into 0.46 percent of total health care spending). The authors present evidence that a combination of factors have contributed to the most recent medical malpractice "crisis," including increased claims costs and decreased investment returns to the insurance companies, resulting in the need to raise rates. The effects of these factors vary substantially from state to state.

Does the System Help Injured Patients?

Hope, Patrick A. "Reforming the Medical Professional Liability Insurance System." The American Journal of Medicine 114 (2003): 622–624. This article discusses the current rise in malpractice insurance rates for physicians and the effects on certain medical specialties. High-risk specialists, particularly obstetricians and surgeons, are having difficulty finding insurance carriers and/or affording medical malpractice premiums; these high rates are causing doctors to move from those states, creating a shortage of doctors in some geographic areas. In addition, few patients recover damages when a malpractice lawsuit is brought to court; seventy percent of the malpractice cases result in no payment to the plaintiff. One conclusion is that many malpractice cases are unwarranted, but, nonetheless, still impose a substantial financial burden on the health care delivery system.

Public Citizen. "Medical Malpractice Payout Trends 1991–2004: Evidence Shows Lawsuits Haven't Caused Doctors' Insurance Woes." Congress Watch, April 2005. Based on findings from the National Practitioner Data Bank (NPDB), which requires all lawsuits to be recorded, this report argues against the popular idea that the increase in medical malpractice insurance rates is due to an increasing number of settlements from lawsuits. The NPDB data suggests that the total number of malpractice payouts to patients in 2004 (4.91 per 100,000 population) is almost the same as in 1991 (5.41), and that the proportion of multi-million dollar payments, when adjusted for inflation, has decreased over the last decade. The report suggests that the problem is with a small number of physicians (5.5 percent) who generate the most malpractice claims (57.3 percent).

Cornell, Emily V. "Addressing the Medical Malpractice Crisis." National Governors' Association, December 5, 2002 (http://www.nga.org). This issue brief discusses the effects of increasing medical malpractice premiums on physicians and medical specialties across specific states in the U.S. Between

2001 and 2002, insurance premiums doubled or tripled in some states, particularly in high-risk specialties such as obstetrics, and, as a result, some health care practitioners began refusing to perform certain procedures. The brief outlines insurance market changes (such as state subsidies), various tort reforms (including damage caps), and legal alternatives (such as mediation). The report cites one state's attempt to reduce malpractice claims by tying liability protection to the use of established practice guidelines.

Does the System Prevent Future Physician Negligence?

Whitehouse, Kaja. "How Good Is Your Doctor?" The Wall Street Journal, June 18, 2006, accessed at www.wsj.com. This article discusses ways consumers and patients can find good quality health care information through web-based information sources. With regard to helping consumers assess the quality of individual physicians, the author lists several websites, including: www.docboard.org, which directs people to state medical boards; www.healthgrades.com, where reports on disciplinary actions against individual physicians, by state, can be purchased for $12.95 each; and www.ratemds.com, which provides information about specific physicians and patient satisfaction levels.

Zuger, Abigail. "Dissatisfaction with Medical Practice." New England Journal of Medicine Volume 350(1) (2004): 69–75. In this special report on the current state of physician dissatisfaction with the medical profession, the author discusses some of the reasons for the discontent. Based on multiple surveys over a period of ten years, the causes of physician frustration with the practice of medicine include managed care, medical malpractice, unrealistic expectations on the part of patients, lack of time, and loss of authority because of regulatory and health plan burdens. With regard to medical malpractice, the author notes that lawsuits drive a wedge through the patient-physician relationship, and no matter what the outcome, physician-defendants are left with feelings of shame, self-doubt, and a disillusion with their profession that may persist for many years.

Kessler, Daniel. "Impact of Malpractice Reforms on the Supply of Physician Services." JAMA 293(21) (2005): 2618–2625. This study examines the supply of physicians in states with reforms in the tort system such as having caps on payments, and reports that states with tort reform increased physician supply. In states that directly limited malpractice liability, physician supply expanded by 2.4 percent in the study period (1985–2001) compared with states without such reforms.

Congressional Budget Office, "Limiting Tort Liability for Medical Malpractice." January 8, 2004. This report discusses the sharp increase in medical malpractice liability insurance premiums between 2000 and 2002, particularly for certain specialties such as obstetricians/gynecologists (twenty-two percent increase) and general surgeons (thirty-three percent increase), and how these premium increases may cause physicians to stop practicing medicine. The authors cited a study analyzing the experience of five sates that reported access problems because of increased malpractice premiums, and found the greatest access problems in rural areas.

"The American Voice 2004: A Pocket Guide to Issues and Allegations." Issues and Allegations: Medical Malpractice. This article discusses the high cost of malpractice insurance premiums and the effects of the high cost on physician services. According to the report, the Blue Cross-Blue Shield Association states that rising insurance costs have led fifty-six percent of doctors in twelve states to refuse to perform certain high-risk procedures and has caused one-third of the physicians to move their practices to another state.

Todd, James. "Reform of the Health Care System and Professional Liability." New England Journal of Medicine 329(23) (1993): 1733–1735. The author, writing as a spokesperson from the American Medical Association, claims that the climate brought on by fears of lawsuits has four major negative effects on medicine, including: (1) driving a wedge between physicians and patients; (2) causing doctors to avoid performing high-risk procedures; (3) increasing the liability to physicians and their medical staff as mid-level practitioners (physician's assistants, nurse practitioners, and other non-physician practitioners) assume more patient care, and (4) increasing defensive medicine, which the author estimates at costing more than $7 billion per year.

Birbeck, G. L. et al. "Do Malpractice Concerns, Payment Mechanisms, and Attitudes Influence Test-ordering Decisions?" Neurology 62 (2004): 119–121. This survey of 595 U.S. neurologists examined their decision to order tests and tried to evaluate the influence of factors not directly related to the care of the patient on test-ordering decisions. Factors associated with higher test ordering included the need for greater reliance in laboratory and other kinds of tests, higher malpractice concerns, and receiving reimbursement. All of these factors entailed more test ordering, and the level of testing was associated with specific physician characteristics (older and board-certified neurologists ordered fewer tests) and practice situations (in-office testing used more often). In general, according to this survey, and in agreement with AMA data, neurologists overestimate their risk of malpractice exposure.

Klingman, D. et al. "Measuring Defensive Medicine Using Clinical Scenario Surveys." J Health Politics Policy and Law 21(2) (Summer 1996): 185–217. This University of Pennsylvania study evaluated, through clinical scenarios given to physicians, whether physicians ordered tests and procedures primarily because of a fear of defensive medicine. The results suggest that the use of defensive medicine varies across clinical situations, and, in most cases, care of the patient and not malpractice concerns caused the decision. The overall percentage of responses indicating that a procedure or test would be ordered because of fear of malpractice seldom exceeded five percent, and that it is more likely that additional testing reflects a more aggressive medical practice style on the part of certain physicians. The authors concluded that defensive medicine, while present, does not exist to the extent suggested by anecdotal evidence or direct physician surveys.

Glassman, P. A. et al. "Physicians' Personal Malpractice Experiences Are Not Related to Defensive Clinical Practices." J Health Politics Policy and Law 21(2) (Summer 1996): 219–241. This companion article to the one cited above asked whether doctors' own experience with being sued causes them to order more tests and practice defensive medicine. In a survey of 1,540 physicians from four specialty groups (cardiologists, surgeons, obstetrician-gynecologists, and internists), the findings reported that the physician's own experience is not a major factor in ordering tests. Physicians with greater malpractice experience showed no differences in initial treatment or follow-up test recommendations.

Studdert, David M. et al. "Defensive Medicine Among High-Risk Specialist Physicians in a Volatile Malpractice Environment." JAMA 293(21) (2005): 2609–2617. This study surveyed physicians in emergency medicine, general surgery, orthopedic surgery, neurosurgery, OB/GYN, and radiology in the state of Pennsylvania to see if they admittedly practiced defensive medicine. Ninety-three percent of participants said they sometimes or often practiced defensive medicine. Fifty-nine percent of participants said they often ordered more diagnostic tests than were medically indicated, and fifty-two percent said they frequently referred patients to other doctors even though the referrals were not medically necessary. Forty-two percent said that liability concerns forced them to change some practices, including avoiding patients with complex medical problems or who appeared that they might sue. Specialist physicians who lacked confidence in the adequacy of their malpractice coverage to protect them or who feared increasing insurance burdens were more than twice as likely to order unnecessary tests. The authors note that it is often difficult to separate defensive medicine from other factors that influence patient care, such as physicians' desire to meet patients' expectations, preserve trust, and avoid conflict. Efforts to reduce defensive medicine should include using practice guidelines.

Harris Interactive. "*Doctors and Other Health Professionals Report Fear of Malpractice Has a Big, and Mostly Negative, Impact on Medical Practice, Unnecessary Defensive Medicine and Openness in Discussing Medical Errors.*" *2003.* This poll found that doctors admittedly practice defensive medicine, with large numbers of physicians—ninety-four percent—reporting that they personally order more tests, refer more patients, prescribe more medication, and suggest biopsies more often than is necessary because of concerns about malpractice. Almost half of the doctors surveyed have considered leaving their practice because of malpractice liability. Physicians believe that fear of litigation discourages physicians from openly discussing and improving medical errors. Only seventeen percent of doctors have faith in the present legal system while the vast majority (ninety-four percent) favor medical courts.

Trying to Fix a Broken System

McCaughey, Betsy. "*Medical Courts Would Heal Infirmities of Legal System.*" *Investor's Business Daily, July 17, 2003.* McCaughey argues that damage caps are not the answer to the medical malpractice problem in America, because she believes that medical courts, without laymen juries, would be better for malpractice litigation because the current system of using jurors is not working. As evidence, the author cites the Harvard Medical Practice Study that reported only two percent of patients who are harmed by negligent physicians actually file a claim, and eighty percent of the winning cases do not represent medical negligence, but rather high-profile cases that elicited a jury's sympathy. The author believes that medical courts would produce fairer and more consistent verdicts.

"Bipartisan Legislation to Create Special Health Courts Is Introduced in the U.S. Senate." Common Good Press Release, June 30, 2005. This press release discusses the proposed federal bill entitled the Fair and Reliable Medical Justice Act of 2005. This Senate bill would establish medical courts for medical malpractice cases with the aim of improving patient safety. Judges experienced in health care law would work full time in these courts.

Struve, Catherine T. "Improving the Medical Malpractice Litigation Process." Health Affairs 23(4) (2004): 33–41. There is a belief among some legal and medical experts that judges and juries cannot adequately address medical liability issues, and this article makes a case for an administrative system that would replace the current system. The author believes that moving toward a no-fault administrative system for medical malpractice cases may be better than expert panels or courts.

Howard, Philip. "The Best Course of Treatment." The New York Times. February 7, 2006. This author of this article believes that malpractice should be taken out of the regular judiciary system. He believes that the legal system has pitted doctors and patients against each other, and recommends using specialized tribunals with expert judges rather than laymen juries.

Mello, Michelle M. et al. "The New Medical Malpractice Crisis." New England Journal of Medicine 348(23) (2003): 2281–2284. This article discusses how various states and medical specialties are experiencing the "new medical malpractice crisis," involving shortages of specialists and reduced affordability of insurance coverage. The author discusses some of the historical reasons for "new" crisis, and outlines one possible policy intervention: the proposed federal liability reform bill, the Help Efficient, Accessible, Low-Cost, Timely Health Care Act. This act combines a $250,000 cap on non-economic awards along with other reforms. The authors suggest that damage caps alone will not reduce medical errors.

Leape, Lucian L. and John A. Fromson. "Problem Doctors: Is There a System-Level Solution?" Ann Intern Med 144 (2006): 1007–115. The authors point out that poor physician performance failures pose threats to patient welfare and safety and they call for a system-wide, national program with formal systems to monitor physician performance and to identify and correct shortcomings. This effort will require collaboration among physician societies, boards, and hospital regulatory bodies.

CHAPTER 13

What Is Managed Care?

Dudley, R. Adams and Harold S. Luft. "Managed Care in Transition." New England Journal of Medicine 344(14) (2001): 1087–1092. This article describes the history of managed care from the early health maintenance organizations (HMOs) like Kaiser-Permanente in the 1960s and 1970s to the growing networks of Preferred Provider Organizations (PPOs) present today. The article introduces the concepts of capitation, gatekeeping, preauthorization for referrals, utilization reviews, practice guidelines, and disease management, all techniques used by HMOs to reduce care in order to control costs. The authors note that most studies have found no difference in the overall quality of care between HMOs and non-HMOs, although there are real concerns about some managed care practices.

Appleby, Julie and Sharon Silke Carty. "Ailing GM Looks to Scale Back Generous Health Benefits." USA Today June 22, 2005. This article discusses the high cost of providing generous health care benefits to automobile workers and cites Lee Iococca's famous quote made in the early 1990s about health insurance costing more than steel.

Miller, Robert H. and Harold S. Luft. "Does Managed Care Lead to Better or Worse Quality of Care?" Health Affairs 16(5) (1997): 7–25. This paper compares the quality of care in HMOs and in non-HMOs. The authors used thirty-seven studies to determine the quality of care in each type of insurance. The findings suggest that there were no significant quality differences in overall medical care. Although managed care organizations did spend less than the non-managed-care plans, patients were less satisfied with their care management even as they were more satisfied with lower health costs. The authors conclude that generalizing about quality of care in managed care is difficult because of their mixed results.

What Went Wrong?

Kerr, Eve A. et al. "The Influence of Gatekeeping and Utilization Review on Patient Satisfaction." JGIM 14 (1999): 287–296. Managed care policies that limited direct access to specialists or denied patient requests for referrals to specialists are related to lower patient satisfaction. This study examines that relationship and finds that "gatekeeping" arrangements that limit access to specialists increase patients' desire to leave their health plan and decrease the likelihood of recommending the medical group or health plan to a friend.

Angell, Marcia. "The Doctor as Double Agent." Kennedy Institute of Ethics Journal 3 (1993): 279–286. This landmark article discusses the roles of physicians under managed care and coined the term "double agent," which describes physicians' opposing obligations to patients and society. Instead of placing health care practitioners in this ethical bind, the author sends a clear message that asking physicians to become "double agents" will reduce patient-centered care.

Council on Ethical and Judicial Affairs, AMA. "Ethical Issues in Managed Care." JAMA 273(4) (1995): 330–335. This AMA council report states the physician's ethical commitment to the patient, and discusses the specific challenges presented by managed care. Managed care creates a financial conflict of interest between patients and physicians and causes physicians to balance patient welfare against financial gain. The council expressed concern about managed care's financial incentives that could lead to reducing appropriate specialist referrals or to withholding needed care. The council recommends that managed care companies create quality incentives that financially reward appropriate care rather than provide financial incentives to reduce care.

Rodwin, Mark A. "Conflicts in Managed Care." New England Journal of Medicine 332(9) (1995): 604–607. This perspective discusses the opposing roles that physicians have practicing under managed care, and the ways physicians and patients are "managed" through policies that restrict patient choice and what physicians are permitted to do. The author identifies the use of financial incentives, lack of patient choice, and the role of the managed care organization's medical director (to approve or deny services) as particular issues that present conflicts in managed care.

What Happened? The Revolt against Managed Care

Bernard, David B. and David J. Shulkin. "The Media vs. Managed Health Care." Archives of Internal Medicine 158 (1998): 2109–2111. This article discussed the influence of the media on the public's perception of managed care. A review of eighty-five news articles showed that only eight percent viewed HMOs positively, while over sixty percent portrayed HMOs negatively. The majority of the articles were about low quality of care, and low patient satisfaction despite the low cost of care. As a result of their findings, the authors predicted that a backlash against managed care was likely.

Freudenheim, Milt. "Penny-Pinching H.M.O.s Showed Their Generosity in Executive Paychecks." New York Times April 11, 1995. Providing an example of how the media contributed to the backlash against managed care, this article discusses the generous salaries and benefits given to medical directors of managed care organizations at a time when costs were being squeezed out of the health care system with reduced services for patients. Critics of the business practice accused the industry of rewarding higher stock prices over improved health care.

Strunk, Bradley C. et al. "Tracking Health Care Costs: Growth Accelerates Again in 2001." Health Affairs 25 (September 2002): W299-310. This article discusses health insurance premium trends from 1991 to 2002, and tracks the ability of managed care to reduce the growth in price from 11.5 percent in 1991 to 0.5 percent in 1996, only to see premiums rise again to 8.3 percent in 2000 and to 12.7 percent in 2002 as the HMO backlash occurred.

Clancy, Carolyn M. and Howard Brody. "Managed Care: Jekyll or Hyde?" JAMA 273(4) (1995): 338–339. Managed care plans are described as "Jekyll or Hyde" plans in which the first (Jekyll) increases and strengthens the physician-patient relationship while promoting population-based, cost-effective, managed care, and the second (Hyde) primary motive is to contain costs by enrolling healthier populations, rationing care, and denying beneficial treatments. The authors call upon the medical leadership in America to foster the patient-centered "Jekyll" model.

Robinson, James C. "The End of Managed Care." JAMA 285(20) (2001): 2622–2628. The author suggests that managed care was "a partial economic success and a total political failure." The promise of managed care—affordable, comprehensive coverage that stressed preventive care—failed because it limited access to certain services and certain physicians. After a decade of trial and error, these strategies angered everyone, and ultimately failed. This led to the "backlash" against capitation and HMOs, and the introduction of "consumer-driven health care" as the next generation of plans.

Miller, Robert H. and Harold S. Luft. "HMO Plan Performance Update: An Analysis of the Literature, 1997–2001." Health Affairs 21(4) (2002): 63–86. Building on earlier studies looking at the quality of managed care plans, the authors analyze seventy-nine studies published from 1997 to 2001 in order to evaluate the quality of care in HMOs. They focus on access, satisfaction, prevention, and health care spending and use. The findings include: overall quality of care is comparable between HMOs and non-HMOs, although HMOs generally had reduced access to physicians and hospitals compared with non-HMO plans; HMOs had high satisfaction ratings for cost but lower patient satisfaction when it came to physician-patient communication; HMOs performed better in the delivery of preventive services (especially some screenings) but performed less well in providing care to poor patients. Overall, the authors conclude that while HMOs and non-HMOs were roughly comparable in providing quality care, most had not accomplished what the "managed care revolution" promised: changing clinical practices and improving quality of care while containing costs for purchasers and consumers. Instead, there were trade-offs and quality, access, or satisfaction had to be given up in exchange for cost savings.

Himmelstein, David et al. "Quality of Care in Investor-Owned vs. Not-for-Profit HMOs." JAMA 281(2) (1999): 159–163. This article examines the difference in quality of care between for-profit HMOs and not-for profit HMOS. The authors report that HMOs, in general, do not seem to have significant differences in the quality of care compared with non-HMOs, except HMOs have worse outcomes with certain vulnerable populations like the poor and the mentally ill. However, for-profit HMOs have significantly lower quality results than not-for-profit HMOs, and for-profit HMOs made up eighty-one percent of the market. Not-for-profit HMOs had better patient compliance, cost less, and had greater preventative care. The authors believe that profits were more important than providing quality care in for-profit HMOs.

Lee, Jason S. and Laura Tollen. "How Low Can You Go? The Impact of Reduced Benefits and Increased Cost Sharing." Health Affairs Web Exclusive (June 19, 2002): W229-241. After a decade of growth in health care spending less than ten percent per year, the managed care backlash ushered in escalating costs once again in 2001, when health insurance premiums grew eleven percent. The authors of this article discuss the cost-control methods from the pre-managed-care era (for example, increased cost sharing by the patient) and suggest that these efforts may provide tools to control health care spending.

Grumbach, Kevin et al. "Primary Care Physicians' Experience of Financial Incentives in Managed-Care Systems." New England Journal of Medicine (Nov 19, 1998): 1516–1521. This article examines the financial incentives that physicians face under managed care to keep costs down. A survey of California physicians revealed that managed care organizations used various types of incentives to influence how physicians practice. Forty percent of physicians reported pressure from managed care organizations' incentives, and many said they believed such pressure decreased the quality of care they were able to provide. Incentives that were based upon quality measures or patient satisfaction were associated with greater job satisfaction among physicians.

Kaiser Family Foundation. "Employer Health Benefits 2004 Annual Survey." http://www.kff.org. This annual report provides statistics about health plan enrollment, insurance premium growth, and other trends in employer health benefits. Between the years of 1996 and 2004, for example, HMO enrollment went down from thirty-one percent to twenty-five percent of those with insurance, while preferred provider organization (PPO) enrollment grew from twenty-eight percent to fifty-five percent.

Kassirer, Jerome. "Managed Care and the Morality of the Marketplace." New England Journal of Medicine. 333(1) (1995): 50–52. This editorial discusses the positive characteristics of the managed care model, including shorter hospital stays, attention to preventive care, the use of evidence-based medicine, and opportunities to measure and encourage quality of care. However, the author also acknowledges that managed care designs have the potential to anger physicians, and cause patients to mistrust physicians.

CHAPTER 14

Holes in the Health Coverage Safety Net

"U.S. Census Bureau News." U.S. Census Bureau August 30, 2005. http://www.census.gov. This article gives a profile of the uninsured, the U.S. population, and the poor. In 2004, eighty-four percent of Americans had health coverage, and sixteen percent (forty-six million) of the population was without health coverage, with almost sixty percent of Americans covered by employer-based insurance, seven percent purchasing health insurance as individuals, and government health programs covering twenty-seven percent (these percentages add up to more than 100 percent because some individuals participated in more than one program during the year). Over eight million children were uninsured. About thirteen percent of all Americans are living at 100 percent of the Federal Poverty Level or below.

Kaiser Commission on Medicaid and the Uninsured. "The Uninsured: A Primer—Key Facts about Americans without Health Insurance." Kaiser Family Foundation January 2006. The report provides an overview of how Americans obtain insurance, describes the uninsured population, and discusses how lack of insurance affects access to health services. The report also reviews public and private insurance programs and their role in reducing the number of Americans without health coverage.

National Health Policy Forum. "Medicare Modernization Act of 2003: Overview of Part D." December 2004. This is an overview of the prescription drug benefit within the federal Medicare program, called "Medicare Part D." The article reviews the benefits, out-of-pocket costs, premiums, deductibles, and low-income assistance associated with the new plan.

Kaiser Family Foundation. "Medicare Spending and Financing." April 2005. http://www.kff.org. This fact sheet is a brief two-page publication that describes Medicare spending, including sources of payment for medical services as well as spending and the Medicare-D drug benefit. Medicare pays less than half of the $11,714 total medical expenditures per individual, while individuals pay nineteen percent of care out-of-pocket, and Medicaid and private insurance (for those who have it) pick up the remaining thirty percent. Ten percent of those covered by Medicare account for sixty-nine percent of the spending. It is projected that Medicare will cover seventy-eight million people by 2030 and that its health insurance trust fund reserves (that pay a large proportion of Medicare) will be exhausted by 2020. The country faces a serious policy challenge: Medicare's financial stability over the long term as it continues to meet the care needs of an aging population.

National Health Policy Forum. "The Basics: Medicare." May 18, 2005. This report gives an overview of Medicare, including enrollment eligibility, services covered, and services not covered. In 2004, about half of Medicare revenues came from payroll taxes, 31.8 percent came from general revenues, and individual premiums represented only 10.5 percent. Currently, forty-two million Americans are covered with total spending of $325 billion.

Kaiser Commission on Medicaid and the Uninsured. "Medicaid Enrollment and Spending Trends." Facts. June 2005. http://www.kff.org. In 2003, Medicaid financed health care for over fifty million low-income children, adults, and elderly and disabled individuals at a total cost of $276 billion. Between 2002 and 2003, Medicaid enrollment increased as a result of economic conditions that made more people eligible for Medicaid as their incomes decreased and many lost employer-sponsored health coverage. At the same time, states attempted to contain costs through a reduction in covered services, as well as requiring those people covered to pay more ("cost sharing"), and through reduced reimbursements to providers.

Kaiser Commission on Medicaid and the Uninsured. "The Medicaid Program at a Glance." Key Facts. January 2005. http://www.kff.org. Medicaid covers more then fifty million people, and the federal government contributes between fifty and seventy-seven percent of Medicaid costs, depending on a state's per-capita income. On average, the federal government financed fifty-seven percent of care. Medicaid covers twenty-five million children, fourteen million adults, five million seniors, and eight million persons with disabilities. The elderly, who make up about twenty-five percent of the population, use more than two-thirds of the benefits. Almost half of Medicaid spending goes toward services for the aged who are eligible for Medicare and Medicaid (the "dual eligibles"). Medicaid finances forty-three percent of long-term care spending, and covers nearly sixty percent of nursing home residents.

Kaiser Family Foundation. "FMAP for Medicaid and Multiplier." http://www.statehealthfacts.org. Each state has a federal matching rate (Federal Medical Assistance Percentage, or FMAP) for the Medicaid program, which determines the ratio of federal/state spending for Medicaid services. The lower per capita income states receive the higher federal match. This fact sheet lists the FMAP rate for the years 2004, 2005, and 2006. Mississippi receives the highest federal match at seventy-six percent in 2006, with California, Colorado, Connecticut, Maryland, Massachusetts, Minnesota, New Hampshire, New York, Virginia, and Washington all receiving the lowest FMAP rate at fifty percent.

Fisher, Gordon M. "The Development and History of the U.S. Poverty Thresholds—A Brief Overview." Department of Health and Human Services (Winter 1997): 6–7. http://www.aspe.hhs.gov/poverty/papers/hptgssiv .htm. This summary explains the development of the poverty threshold in the United States, commonly known as the "Federal Poverty Level" (FPL). Molly Orshansky of the Social Security Administration determined the FPL in 1963. She based her calculations on the Department of Agriculture's "economy food plan," a nutritionally adequate, but extremely inexpensive food plan that would be used during times of financial hardship. Families of three or more spent about thirty percent of their after-tax income on food in 1955. In determining the FPL, Orshansky multiplied the cost of the economy food plan by three. Orshansky presented the poverty threshold as a measure of inadequate income, stating, "If it is not possible to state unequivocally 'how much is enough,' it should be possible to assert with confidence how much, on average, is too little." There have been many recommendations to change the way the U.S. measures poverty, but none has replaced this original calculation.

Wessel, David. "Counting the Poor: Methods and Controversy." The Wall Street Journal, June 15, 2006, page A10. This report on poverty in the U.S. describes how the U.S. measures poverty, what is meant by the "Federal Poverty Line," and how many Americans are poor today. Families whose incomes fall under a poverty threshold or "Federal Poverty Line" are considered poor, and the poverty line varies by family size. In 2004, although almost thirteen percent of the U.S. population was poor (thirty-seven million), children (17.8 percent of all children) and blacks (24.7 percent of blacks) disproportionately represent the poor.

For more information about the U.S. Poverty Guidelines, go to: http:// aspe.hhs.gov/poverty/06poverty.shtml.

The Kaiser Commission on Medicaid and the Uninsured. "SCHIP Program Enrollment: June 2003 Update." Prepared by Vernon K. Smith and David M. Rousseau, December 2003. This report, based on data provided by the State Children's Health Insurance Program (SCHIP) and Medicaid officials, outlines current SCHIP enrollment, variation by state and SCHIP program type, and program changes. The publication lists the states that cover adults as part of their SCHIP program as well as those states that have caps on the number of enrollees, premiums, or enrollment fees.

Information about the Veterans Administration's medical benefits can be accessed at: http://www1.va.gov/opa/fact/vafacts.html.

Why There Are So Many Uninsured Despite Public Programs

Steinberg, Marc. "Working without a Net: The Health Care Safety Net Still Leaves Millions of Low-Income Workers Uninsured." Families USA, April 2004. Using U.S. Census Bureau data, this "special report" indicates that fourteen million low-income adults do not qualify for public health programs or have employer-sponsored health insurance despite the fact that they work. More than sixty-two percent of all uninsured workers were either self-employed or working in small businesses with fewer than 100 employees. Some states have expanded access to address the health insurance needs of this population, using waivers from the federal government to allow states to raise their Medicaid income levels or using unspent SCHIP funds. Some programs have faced restrictions such as caps, or are already frozen at their current size. Examples of such coverage expansions include Tennessee subsidized care for adults below 400 percent of the Federal Poverty Level, but had to cap the program in 1995 because of the high demand. Illinois expanded coverage for parents up to 185 percent of the federal poverty level.

Dubay, Lisa and Genevieve Kenney. "Addressing Coverage Gaps for Low-Income Parents." 23(2) (2004): 225–234. This article examines how rates of uninsurance for low-income parents could be reduced using state-level initiatives. States have the option of creating health coverage programs for low-income parents through either SCHIP or as a Medicaid expansion. If state governments covered all parents up to 200 percent of the Federal Poverty Level, 7.4 million adults would qualify for the insurance. However, fiscal problems in the states do not permit generous expansions for low-income parents, and, to that end, the authors conclude that 100 percent federal funding (without requiring the states to match any funds) may be needed to reduce the coverage gaps among low-income populations.

Center on Budget and Policy Priorities. "Expanding Medicaid Coverage to Low-Income Parents Reduces Number of Uninsured Children, New Research Finds." September 5, 2000. Although ninety percent of children from low-income families are eligible for Medicaid or SCHIP, many low-income children—up to twenty-five percent of them—remain uninsured. Part of the reason for this insurance gap, according to this study, is the ineligibility of the children's parents for public insurance. In looking at Medicaid expansions that included health coverage for parents, the study reported that the number of low-income children protected by health insurance also increased as a result of their parents' coverage. Comparing changes in children's coverage in states that had coverage for low-income parents with states that did not, the authors conclude that allowing an entire family to apply for health insurance increases the likelihood that children will also be covered.

Kaiser Commission on Medicaid and the Uninsured. "Enrolling Low-Income Children in Medicaid and SCHIP." Fact Sheet, March 2005. www.kff.org. This 2005 fact sheet reports that in 2002 there were ten million children in the U.S. without health coverage and that sixty-two percent, 6.2 million children, were eligible for either Medicaid (forty-five percent) or SCHIP (fifty-five percent). The authors suggest that states' financial problems and administrative burdens have led to enrollment barriers.

Guendelman, Sylvia and Michelle Pearl. "Children's Ability to Access and Use Health Care." Health Affairs 23(2) (2004): 235–244. This article describes the use of federal "waivers" (allowing exceptions in Medicaid rules) to extend the public programs to low-income families (and not just children). California, Connecticut, the District of Columbia, and New York have used waivers to provide health coverage for low-income parents. Earlier studies suggest that these kinds of expansions for parents help stimulate higher enrollment for young children.

Weil, Alan. "There's Something about Medicaid." Health Affairs 22(1) (2003): 13–29. This article states that Medicaid suffers from a mismatch between what we ask it to do and what we are willing to pay to support the program. Medicaid pays for one-third of all childbirths and insures one out of five children. Medicaid is the largest payer for AIDS patients and also provides payments to community health centers, safety-net hospitals, and mental health systems. Although enrollment in Medicaid has grown from four million in 1966 to forty-seven million in 2002, not everyone who is eligible enrolls in the program, often because it is neither easy nor convenient to enroll; only seventy-two percent of eligible children and fifty-one percent of eligible non-elderly adults are enrolled. This suggests that the program could grow by more than twenty million (to over seventy million) children and non-elderly adults if all who were eligible enrolled. Medicaid programs increase and decrease with the economic status of state budgets, adding and subtracting "optional" low-income populations as revenues change. The author concludes that the funding and coverage "roller-coaster" nature of Medicaid makes the vital safety net program at risk.

Nolan, Lea et al. "Enrolling Uninsured Children in SCHIP." Journal of Ambulatory Care Management. 26(1) (2003): 51–62. This article looks at the role that community heath centers (CHCs) play in enrolling children in public insurance programs. Thirty percent of the children who receive care at CHCs are uninsured. Despite efforts at fourteen CHCs in six states, there were small gains in enrollment, which the authors blame on state eligibility policies, potential enrollees' lack of awareness of the programs, and difficult application procedures.

Feder, Judith et al. "Covering the Low-Income Uninsured: The Case for Expanding Public Programs." Health Affairs (January 2001): 27–39. This author argues for strengthening the health coverage safety net for the low-income uninsured population who can least afford private insurance. Specific reforms would include expanding public health programs and removing the barriers in the existing programs, including long application procedures, tests of family assets, and requirements to reenroll as often as every six months, all of which require a great deal of paperwork. She concludes that it will take a variety of strategies to address the problems of extending coverage to all of the uninsured; for those with the lowest incomes, public programs need to be strengthened and expanded.

Spencer, Anna. "Community Health Centers: Serving the Nation's Most Vulnerable Populations." National Conference of State Legislatures. February 23, 2004. Community health centers (CHCs) deliver care to low-income populations. In 2002, there were more than 3,500 centers serving over fourteen million people, the majority of whom had incomes below 200 percent of the Federal Poverty Level. CHCs provide services that increase immunizations, provide prenatal care, alleviate health problems and lower Medicaid costs. More than sixty percent of CHC patients are minorities, eighty-six percent earn less than 200 percent of the Federal Poverty Level, forty percent lack health insurance, and one-third speak a first language other than English. CHCs save the Medicaid program thirty percent per beneficiary each year, totaling $3 billion in annual savings for federal and state governments.

Cunningham, Peter and Jack Hadley. "Expanding Care versus Expanding Coverage: How to Improve Access to Care." Health Affairs 23(4) (2004): 234–244. This article examines the two primary ways to increase access to care for the low-income uninsured: through expanding public insurance coverage and through increased funding for community health centers. CHCs serve the uninsured but must meet certain requirements to locate in areas with a specific low ratio of doctors to population ("medically underserved" areas), whereas insurance expansions can be more flexible. Greater CHC funding may increase access to care, but CHCs do not provide specialty care services or reduce the use of hospital emergency rooms. The authors conclude that insurance expansions and CHC expansions must be used together to increase coverage for the low-income uninsured.

Getting Worse

Hadley, Jack et al. "Federal Spending on the Health Care Safety Net from 2001–2004: Has Spending Kept Pace with the Growth in the Uninsured?" Executive Summary. Kaiser Family Foundation. November 2005. Federal spending is the largest component of funding for the uninsured, providing an estimated $20 billion in funding in 2001. Total federal spending grew by 15.4 percent between 2001 and 2004, and federal support for community health centers grew by fifty percent. However, adjusting for inflation, total federal spending only increased by 1.3 percent between 2001 and 2004, and, at the same time, the number of the uninsured grew by 11.2 percent. As a result, federal spending per uninsured person actually deceased by 8.9 percent, suggesting that federal support for the uninsured has not kept pace with the increase in the number of uninsured Americans.

Gilmer, Todd and Richard Kronick. "It's the Premiums, Stupid: Projections of the Uninsured through 2013." Health Affairs (April 5, 2005): W5-143-151. This article predicts that the number of uninsured will grow to fifty-six million by 2013; for every one-percent increase in health spending, relative to personal income, 246,000 people will lose health insurance. The authors conclude that our current system of employer-sponsored health insurance (or any other alternative system) cannot continue without more successful cost containment efforts.

CHAPTER 15

Uninsured and Working

Kaiser Commission on Medicaid and the Uninsured. "The Uninsured: A Primer—Key Facts About Americans Without Health Insurance." Kaiser Family Foundation. January 2006. The twenty-five-page report provides an overview of how Americans obtain insurance, describes the uninsured population, and discusses how lack of insurance affects access to health care. Over eighty percent of the uninsured come from working families. The report also reviews public and private insurance programs and their role in reducing the number of Americans without health insurance coverage.

The Kaiser Family Foundation and Health Research and Educational Trust. "Employer Health Benefits: 2005 Summary of Findings." 2005. This annual survey of private and public employers presents current information about employer-sponsored health insurance in the U.S. Employer-sponsored health insurance provides coverage for 160 million Americans, protecting nearly three out of five Americans under the age of sixty-five. This report includes information about the number of firms offering health insurance by size, the average premium cost by plan/single/family, and small-firm premiums compared to large-firm premiums. Deductibles are usually higher in small firms rather than in large firms because the overall health insurance premium is higher for small businesses who have fewer employees to spread the financial risk. The report compares the average premiums for High Deductible Health Plans and Health Savings Accounts.

Dorn, Stan. "Towards Incremental Progress: Key Facts about Groups of Uninsured." Economic and Social Research Institute, September 2004. The report presents categories of uninsured Americans who could benefit from incremental health coverage expansions. These categories include employees of small businesses, workers who lose their jobs, workers who refuse employer coverage, low-income parents, low-income childless adults, the near-elderly (fifty-five to sixty-five years old), young adults, children, and immigrants. Along with each fact sheet is an analysis of the types of health policy changes that could encourage health coverage. Some of the key information that provides targets for these policies include: nearly half of the uninsured are either self-employed or work at firms with fewer than twenty-five workers; most uninsured workers (sixty percent) have employers that do not provide health insurance; twenty-two percent are offered employer coverage but refuse it, mainly because of cost; one-third of low-income parents lack health insurance. Once older Americans lose coverage they are much more likely to remain uninsured (twenty-two percent versus twelve percent for other younger populations measured over a four-year period) and young adults between the ages of nineteen and twenty-nine are the largest group of the uninsured, representing thirty percent, even though they make up only seventeen percent of those under sixty-five.

The Insurance Market for Individuals

Bernard, Didem M. "Premiums in the Individual Health Insurance Market for Policyholders under Age 65, 1996 and 2002." Statistical Brief No. 72. AHRQ March 2005. This statistical brief compares individual insurance rates and premiums between 1996 and 2002. In 2002, 4.8 percent of the U.S. population under the age of sixty-five (12.1 million) had individual health insurance, compared with sixty-nine percent (174 million people) who held employer-based coverage. The average individual premium in 2002 was $1,913 for single coverage (with the 90th percentile at $4,728) and the average premium was $4227 for family coverage (with the 90th percentile at $7481). In 1996 and 2002, seventy percent of individual policies were purchased for single people, and thirty percent were for families. There is great variation in benefit and deductibles as well as "medical underwriting," which determines who is denied access to insurance because of health status or pre-existing conditions. Older people pay higher premiums than younger people.

Kaiser Family Foundation and eHealthInsurance. "Update on Individual Health Insurance," August 2005. The report gives an overview of the differences in premiums based on age, geographic region, and benefit level. Family purchasers are usually older than single purchasers, and younger people keep their policies for a shorter amount of time because they are often between jobs or just entering the workforce. According to their tables, a family policy with a $1,500 deductible would cost, on average, $281 per month but with high deductibles and limited benefits. The authors note that the large difference between the average costs of individually purchased coverage compared with group health insurance offered by larger employers likely is due to the relatively younger ages of individual health insurance purchasers and less generous coverage, which may not cover all of the purchaser's health care needs, but may provide just enough to keep insurance affordable.

Buntin, Melinda Beeuwkes et al. "The Role of the Individual Health Insurance Market and Prospects for Change." Health Affairs 23(6) (2004): 79–89. The individual health insurance market is the only source of health insurance for the more than one out of five Americans who are not eligible for group or public health insurance. This article discusses how the demand for individual policies is affected by high prices, citing how in California persons earning below 200 percent of the Federal Poverty Level would have to pay almost fifteen percent of their income on premiums, and sick people would have to pay even more. However, despite the problems in the individual health insurance market, there are advantages as well: individual coverage is relatively affordable for those who want to insure against only catastrophic medical accidents. The authors conclude that growth in the mobility of the American workforce will create a greater demand for the purchase of individual health insurance, but unless and until public policies are developed to balance affordability with availability to those other than the healthy, the individual insurance market will not be effective in expanding health coverage overall.

Turnbull, Nancy C. and Nancy M. Kane. "Insuring the Healthy or Insuring the Sick? The Dilemma of Regulating the Individual Health Insurance Market." The Commonwealth Fund, February 2005. Health insurance policies purchased in the individual market are frequently not available or the premiums are so high as to be unaffordable to those with preexisting health conditions—those who need insurance the most. This report examines how state regulations in seven states have affected overall health coverage in those states, and concludes that in the current system there will always be the tradeoff between affordability and availability, with suppliers of insurance avoiding the high-risk population in order to keep the price of insurance down. The only "fix" to this is to require people to have insurance, and this would have a very large pool of people among whom risk would be shared.

Nichols, Len M. *"Challenges Facing Small Employers in Purchasing Health Insurance." A Statement before the U.S. Senate Committee on Small Business and Entrepreneurship, April 20, 2005.* In this testimony, the author cites that forty-four percent of businesses with fewer than fifty workers offer health insurance compared with ninety-seven percent of large businesses, covering sixty-four percent and ninety-eight percent of workers, respectively. This is largely due to the ability of larger companies to take advantage of economies of scale, and having large "risk pools," for example, large numbers of employees to spread the risk.

Gencarelli, Dawn M. *"Health Insurance Coverage for Small Employers." NHPF Background Paper, April 19, 2005.* This background paper discusses the concerns of workers in small businesses surrounding the affordability of health insurance and examines the problems facing these workers and their employers. Small firms usually have workers who are paid less, have less education, and work part time; therefore, small businesses have a greater proportion of low income workers who are also less able to afford the health insurance premiums. The author notes that despite years of state and federal efforts, health insurance premiums continue to rise in the small-group market faster than in the large employer market.

Gabel, J. et al. *"Generosity and Adjusted Premiums in Job-Based Insurance: Hawaii Is Up, Wyoming Is Down." Health Affairs 25(3) (2006): 832–843.* This study reports national and state findings on the actuarial value of U.S. employer-based plans, and their adjusted premiums, in 2002. After adjusting for the quality of the benefits, the authors find that health insurance premiums are eighteen percent higher in the nation's smallest firms (one to nine workers) than in firms with 1,000 or more workers.

Ditsler, Elaine et al. *"On the Fringe: The Substandard Benefits of Workers in Part-Time, Temporary, and Contract Jobs." The Commonwealth Fund, December 2005.* About twenty-five percent of the U.S. workforce is made up of people in "non-standard" jobs, such as the self-employed, part-time workers, independent contractors, and temporary workers, and they have limited access to employer-sponsored health insurance. They are twice as likely as full-time workers to be uninsured; they are five times more likely to rely on public programs, and they are more than three times as likely to rely on a spouse for coverage. Although forty percent of non-standard workers are offered health insurance (compared with eighty-seven percent of full-time workers), only fifty-four percent of them (compared with eighty-five percent of full-time workers) "take up" the offered insurance. As a result, only fifteen percent of children and sixteen percent of spouses have health insurance through the non-standard worker's employer.

How Much Can People Afford?

Kaiser Commission on Medicaid and the Uninsured, "Challenges and Tradeoffs in Low-Income Family Budgets: Implications for Health Coverage," April 2004. This report, based on interviews of twelve families in three cities in 2003, records the experiences of low-income families balancing household expenses and needs, looking at the financial pressures and choices. Low-income families spend seven out of ten dollars on basic living expenses such as housing (thirty-three percent), transportation (twenty percent), and food (seventeen percent), with health care accounting for up to seven percent of the family budget, and frequently less. Although the study involved twelve low-income families at varying stages of life, there were some common themes among the families: 1) family finances are uncertain, and many live paycheck to paycheck with little savings and increasing debt, resulting in fear of poor credit ratings; 2) almost none of the families had employer-sponsored health insurance, and many families, even those few with employer-sponsored coverage, report they have large unpaid medical bills from unexpected medical problems, making them reluctant to seek needed care in the future; and 3) many families reported that they would welcome public health coverage such as Medicaid and SCHIP, but most do not want cash assistance, i.e., welfare.

Long, Sharon K. "Hardship among the Uninsured: Choosing among Food, Housing, and Health Insurance." The Urban Institute, New Federalism, Series B, No. B-54, May 2003. In this analysis of findings from the National Survey of America's Families, researchers note that for many low-income uninsured adults, the decision to purchase health insurance competes with demands for basic food and housing. Previous studies have suggested that when premiums exceed five percent of income for low-income individuals, less people buy health insurance. The findings from this study detail the consequences: Fifty-seven percent of low-income uninsured adults faced food or housing hardship, and thirty-three percent faced the possibility of high insurance costs because of health problems. The researchers suggest that efforts to increase health insurance coverage must take into account the competing demands of other household expenses on the limited resources of low-income individuals and families.

Wertheimer, Richard. "Poor Families in 2001: Parents Working Less and Children Continue to Lag Behind." Child Trends Research Brief, No. 2003-10, May 2003. This paper reports statistics on health insurance coverage and child care services among poor families during the recession of 2001: working poor two-parent families spent as much as twenty-three percent of their income on child care and children in low-income families were less likely to be covered by health insurance.

Davis, Karen et al. "How High Is Too High? Implications of High-Deductible Health Plans." The Commonwealth Fund, publication No. 816, April 2005. This report suggests that high-deductible health plans (HDHPs) are not a viable option for low-income adults because people with incomes below $35,000 using a HDHP would: a) experience serious financial problems (forty-four percent compared with twenty-one percent of higher-income, insured adults); b) have more medical bill problems (fifty-four percent compared with twenty-four percent); and c) if chronically ill, fifty-nine percent of HDHP-enrollees would build up medical debt compared with twenty-four percent of the chronically ill in health plans with lower deductibles. The authors state that the major effect of HDHPs would be to shift spending from insurance premiums to out-of-pocket spending, which will create financial hardship for low-income individuals and families. Two-thirds of the uninsured have incomes that are less than 200 percent of the Federal Poverty Level, and premiums for HDHPs for virtually all the uninsured are more than five percent of income—the best would be for a twenty-five-year-old living male at two hundred percent the Federal Poverty Level—but still six percent of income, but for a sixty-year old woman at the same income level, it would be around twenty percent of income.

Merlis, M. et al. "Rising Out-of-Pocket Spending for Medical Care: A Growing Strain on Family Budgets." The Commonwealth Fund publication number 887, February 2006. In 2001–2002, nearly forty-three percent of families spent between five and ten percent of total income on health care and eighteen percent of families had health care costs greater than ten percent of income. Family health care expenses are getting worse: employee contributions toward family premiums have increased twenty-seven percent between 2002 and 2005, suggesting that this trend of higher health spending relative to family income will continue and that families will continue to contribute a growing share of their budgets to health care costs. This may increase the numbers of the uninsured or increase the level of medical debt, particularly among low-income families.

Fronstin, Paul. "The Relationship Between Income and Health Insurance: Rethinking the Use of Family Income in the Current Population Survey." EBRI Notes. 26(2) (2005). This article focuses on higher income families that do not have health insurance. Using estimates from the 2004 Current Population Survey, eleven million uninsured individuals, accounting for twenty-five percent of the uninsured, are in families with incomes of $50,000 or more, with seven percent of the uninsured in families with incomes of greater than $75,000 a year. About four million of the eleven million "high-income uninsured" are either adult children who are not full-time students but continue living with their parents, and over eighty percent of the 3.9 million earn less than $50,000 per year. Only 4.7 million are either the head of the family or the spouse of the head of the family, with two million children, grandchildren, and other relatives under the age of eighteen. In looking at the total distribution of Americans under the age of sixty-five without health insurance by family income, forty-seven percent have family incomes of less than $25,000/year.

Schoen, Cathy, et al. "Insured But Not Protected: How Many Adults Are Underinsured?" Health Affairs Web Exclusive (June 14, 2005): W5-289-W5-302. In addition to the forty-five million uninsured persons in the U.S. in 2003, this study finds that there were sixteen million additional Americans who were "underinsured," defined as having health insurance that would not cover them adequately if their health treatment became costly. Underinsured individuals are almost as likely to go without needed care as uninsured individuals. People are underinsured if they fall under one of the three criteria: annual out-of-pocket expenses are greater than ten percent or more of family income; incomes are less than two hundred percent of the Federal Poverty Level and out-of-pocket health care expenses are greater than five percent of income; and health plan deductibles are more than five percent of income. In this study, nearly sixteen million were underinsured in 2003, with seventy-three percent of the sixteen million having annual incomes below two hundred percent of the Federal Poverty Level. Along with the forty-five million Americans who went without health coverage all or part of the year, a total of sixty-one million were either underinsured or uninsured in 2003.

Collins, S. R. et al. "Gaps in Health Insurance: An All-American Problem." The Commonwealth Fund, April 2006. This report discusses the growing problem of obtaining and keeping health insurance, even for those Americans who are not considered low-income. Forty-one percent of adults with incomes between $20,000 and $40,000 a year did not have health insurance for at least part of 2005, up from twenty-eight percent in 2001. More than half of the nearly 4,500 people expressed difficulty paying medical bills despite the fact that most of them had health insurance; more than one-third of the 4,500 people reported problems or delays in going to the doctor because of cost.

Wicks, Elliot K. et al. "Tax Options to Promote the Purchase of Health Insurance." Economic and Social Research Institute. August 2004. This brief was prepared for the state of Maryland and offers tax options to promote the purchase of health insurance. One of the options recommended is to adopt a tax penalty for high-income residents who fail to purchase health insurance coverage. Penalty thresholds could be set at the state average income ($55,900 in 2003), or indexed to the Federal Poverty Level at 400 percent (approximately $63,000). These families would be required to pay a penalty unless they can demonstrate they and their children have health coverage for at least seventy-five percent of the year. They argue that the absence of insurance coverage creates problems for the rest of the state, including higher private and public spending to compensate for the care.

For more information about the April 2006 health coverage reform plan in Massachusetts, which requires individuals to have health insurance or pay a penalty, see: http://www.kff.org/uninsured/upload/7494.pdf.

CHAPTER 16

A Quirk of History

Healthcare Leadership Council. "This Health Insurance Guide Is for You." Cover the Uninsured Week 2005, May 2005, http://covertheuninsured.org/. This is a guide for individuals, the self-employed, and small employers looking for health insurance for themselves or for their employees. As part of the materials issued every year in the Robert Wood Johnson Foundation program, "Cover the Uninsured Week," the guide discusses the types and costs of health insurance and gives examples about how offering health insurance reduces worker turnover, and provides beneficial tax advantages. The cost of health insurance with tax advantages can provide up to a forty-percent savings to employers, which markedly reduces the cost of purchasing insurance.

Insure.com. HIPAA: Your Rights to Health Insurance Portability, 2003, http://www.insure.com. This article gives an overview of the federal Health Insurance Portability and Accountability Act (HIPAA), passed in 1996; one of the purposes of the act is to address an employment problem known as "job lock": a condition in which employees are reluctant to change jobs for fear of losing health insurance benefits. HIPAA prevents companies from withholding health insurance for preexisting conditions provided that the worker had group health insurance for at least twelve months prior to changing jobs and that the new job offers group coverage. HIPAA also provides that if an employee had health insurance continuously in the previous job, if the new employer provides health insurance, then the new company must offer insurance without a waiting period. However, the new company may charge a great deal more for that coverage.

Pros and Cons of the Employer-Based System

Kaiser Family Foundation. "Employer Health Benefits: 2005 Annual Survey." Exhibit 2.6 (page 37) reports that forty-three percent of the employers surveyed list "administrative hassles" as very important or somewhat important in deciding not to offer health insurance as an employee benefit.

Mulvey, Janemarie. "Rising Benefit Costs Crowd Out Wage Growth." Employment Policy Foundation, March 31, 2005. This fact sheet examines the relationship between growth rates in employer health insurance costs and employee wages. Over the past twenty years, employer health care costs have doubled as a percentage of average wages from 5.5 percent in 1984 to 11.6 percent in 2004. Health insurance was the largest employer-provided benefit in 2004, accounting for almost a third of all benefits. Manufacturing and transportation sectors have been hardest hit from rising health care costs.

The Leapfrog Group. http://www.leapfroggroup.org. The Leapfrog Group is a group of more than 170 employer organizations that purchase health care for more than thirty-seven million people in the US. Leapfrog takes advantage of its purchasing power to initiate "big leaps" in health care safety, quality, and affordability for its members, which they accomplish by awarding contracts and giving rewards to hospitals who meet quality and safety standards and practices. Leapfrog's thirty-one regions encompass almost 2,000 urban, suburban, and rural hospitals, and Leapfrog officials state that their quality and safety practices have the potential to save up to 65,342 lives and prevent up to 907,600 medication errors each year.

Fronstin, Paul. "Source of Health Insurance and Characteristics of the Uninsured: Analysis of the March 2005 Current Population Survey." Employee Benefit Research Institute, Issue Brief No. 287, November 2005. This report analyzes and summarizes the U.S. Census Bureau's March 2005 Current Population Survey (CPS). In 2004, overall health insurance coverage continued to decline, with employment-based coverage dropping. The analysis reports that employment status remains the most important determinant of health insurance coverage, with large employers able to provide health benefits at lower cost than small employers (because they are subject to less adverse selection and their administrative costs are lower) and, therefore, workers in large firms are more likely to be covered than those in small firms. Most of the uninsured work in small businesses where health insurance is less available and more expensive to the worker.

Kaiser Family Foundation. "Employer Health Benefits: 2005 Summary of Findings." Publication No. 7316, 2005. Employer-sponsored health insurance provides coverage for 160 million Americans, covering nearly sixty percent of those under sixty-five. This survey summary reports on changes in health insurance premiums for workers, amounts employees have to pay, availability of employer-based coverage, health plan enrollment figures, and the use of high-deductible health plans. Although growth in health insurance premiums has lessened slightly in recent years, it continues to increase faster than general inflation and wages. Over the last five years, health insurance premiums have grown by seventy-three percent compared with general inflation of fourteen percent and wage growth of fifteen percent. The percentage of small firms offering health benefits fell from sixty-three percent to fifty-nine percent between 2003 and 2004, compared with ninety-nine percent and ninety-eight percent of large firms. Average deductibles are higher for small firms than for large firms, although all employers are requiring employees to pay more of the cost. The report states that about twenty percent of firms now offer high-deductible health plans (HDHPs).

The Robert Wood Johnson Foundation. "Why Should Policy-Makers Care?" Policy Brief, No. 7, December 2005. This brief examines the reasons why employers decide to offer health coverage and how employers will respond to private and public policy initiatives to increase health insurance coverage. Businesses that offer health insurance usually have higher wage workers, unionized workers, or are in manufacturing and public sectors. Employers who are unlikely to offer coverage are those whose employees are lower wage workers. Previous studies suggest that health insurance costs are shifted to workers in the form of lower wages, although the opposite is rarely seen: when workers do not buy insurance coverage, their wages do not increase.

Not All Businesses Are Equal

Gabel, Jon R., and Jeremy D. Pickreign. "Risky Business: When Mom and Pop Buy Health Insurance for Their Employees." The Commonwealth Fund, publication No. 722, April 2004. Surveys of small businesses show that rapid premium increases are resulting in more of the cost being passed along to the employees. In 2003, premiums for small firms increased over fifteen percent compared with thirteen percent for large firms, and deductibles increased 100 percent for small firms compared with thirty-three percent for larger firms. Almost half of employees in small firms contributed forty-one percent or more of the family health insurance premium compared with only eleven percent in large firms. The authors conclude that fundamental change in the small employer market is necessary.

Headd, Brian. "The Characteristics of Small-Business Employees," Monthly Labor Review (April 2000): 13–18. Small businesses (as defined in this article as having fewer than 500 employees) employ slightly more than half of the private-sector workforce. This comprehensive review of small business includes a look at employees by race, gender, education, age, and occupation. The author reports that small businesses are most likely in the goods and services sectors such as construction, restaurants, agriculture, and fishing. These labor sectors report higher percentages of employees that work part-time, have less education, and are on public assistance. They have lower compensation and less availability of pension and health benefits.

Gencarelli, Dawn M. "Health Insurance Coverage for Small Employers." National Health Policy Forum, Background Paper, April 19, 2005. This report discusses the problems small businesses experience in providing workers with affordable insurance coverage. Small firms usually have workers that are paid less, have less education, and work part time. Smaller employee groups (fewer than 200 employees in this study) have fewer persons among whom to spread risk, making them more vulnerable to high-cost claims even from a few employees. More than seventy-five percent of businesses in the U.S. are considered small; they employ over thirty percent of the private sector workforce. Small firms are more likely to be located in rural areas, represent the goods and service industries, tend to have lower wages, employ more women and minorities, and provide less generous health benefits. The health care administrative costs for small companies are higher than for large companies because health insurance premiums are based on the medical experience of the employees. In addition, many small businesses are not aware of the tax deductions available for health insurance. A survey of small employers in 2002 found that fifty-seven percent of employers surveyed did not know that health insurance premiums were deducted as a business expense. This lack of knowledge, according to the author, may contribute to the lower offer rate of health insurance to employees in small businesses.

Glied, Sherry and Phyllis Borzi. "The Current State of Employment-Based Health Coverage." The Journal of Law, Medicine, and Ethics (Fall 2004): 404–409. This article summarizes the history of the employment-based health coverage system in the U.S., including the origins and rationale of the current system. The advantages of the work-based U.S. health system include favorable tax treatment of coverage for employers and employees, greater health security, and administrative cost advantages, in terms of purchasing a health plan as well as having a larger risk pool in large employers. As a result, the cost of coverage for large businesses is about forty percent lower than for workers who purchased coverage for themselves or their family in the individual market. The criticisms of the voluntary system include the potential for lack of ability to change jobs because of a worker's health status ("job lock"), the high costs of health insurance premiums that may decrease growth in wages, and the restriction of the type of plans available at the workplace. In 2003, forty-seven percent of workers had only one health plan choice through their employer, and these workers were mostly working for small businesses (seventy percent of businesses with fewer than 200 employees only offer just one plan compared with twenty percent of large businesses with more than 5,000 workers). This lack of choice leads some healthy or low-income employees to forgo purchasing health coverage altogether because, despite the group rate, they still find the coverage too expensive. However, despite the drawbacks, the majority of employees, historically as much as two-thirds, prefer employment-based coverage over government or individual coverage, as reported in the 2003 Health Confidence Survey conducted by the Employer Benefit Research Institute (EBRI). The authors conclude that any public policy to expand health insurance coverage would have to take into account the long history of job-based insurance, and that finding an alternative to the current system will be difficult. Despite its flaws, employment-based health insurance is popular with employees, offers affordable rates relative to individual coverage, and is successful in providing health coverage to large numbers of Americans.

U.S. Department of Labor, Occupational Safety and Health Administration. "OSHA Facts—December 2004." http://www.osha.gov/as/opa/oshafacts.html. The current fatality rate while at work is four deaths per 100,000 workers and almost three-quarters of work-related injuries happened in goods-producing or service industries, many of which are small businesses, such as restaurants.

Gabel, Jon R. et al. "Embraceable You: How Employers Influence Health Plan Enrollment." Health Affairs 20(4) (2001): 196–208. Based on a survey of almost 2000 employers, this study examines the policies that affect the percentage of workers eligible and enrolled in a firm's health plan. Workers are more likely to accept coverage when the price is low and when employers offer a choice of plans. The author reports that over eighty percent of workers in small firms have no choice of plans compared with ninety percent of employees in large firms that have more than one choice. Retail businesses have the lowest rates of employees who buy health insurance, while state and local government employees and transportation employees have the highest enrollment rate. The author suggests that health insurance premium prices and employee incomes were the main determinants in health plan enrollment.

CHAPTER 17

A Matter of Life or Death

Institute of Medicine. "Hospital-based Emergency Care: At the Breaking Point." National Academy of Sciences, June 2006. This report discusses the current "epidemic" of overcrowding, lack of available resources, and insufficient capacity facing hospital-based emergency rooms in the U.S. health system. According to the experts conducting the study, U.S. emergency care lacks the capacity to respond to large epidemics or disasters. Half a million times a year, or once every minute, ambulances carrying patients to hospital emergency rooms are turned away and sent to other hospitals farther away because of full emergency rooms. The high demand and overcrowding of hospital emergency rooms comes from several pressures on the system: a reduction of emergency rooms over the last decade, and the increased use of emergency rooms for medical care by Americans who lack health coverage.

Brown, David. "Crisis Seen in Nation's ER Care." Washington Post, June 15, 2006, page A01. This newspaper story announces the release of the Institute of Medicine's (IOM) report on the problems facing the emergency medical care system in the U.S. (see reference No. 1 above). The news item states that people coming to hospital emergency rooms who require inpatient hospital treatment sometimes wait up to two days before an available hospital bed becomes available.

Institute of Medicine. "Care without Coverage: Too Little, Too Late." National Academy of Sciences, May 2002. This report concludes that health insurance is associated with better health outcomes for adults, and the lack of insurance results in greater decreases in health status and premature death. Adults with chronic conditions stand to benefit the most from health insurance coverage because their need for health care is greater. Racial and ethnic minorities, as well as lower-income adults, would particularly benefit from having health insurance because they have worse health status. Uninsured adults have death rates twenty-five percent higher than privately insured persons. The uninsured are at greater risk for premature death because they receive fewer preventive services, and less effective treatment for acute medical conditions. For example, the report finds that uninsured women with breast cancer have a thirty to fifty percent higher risk of dying than insured women, and patients with colon cancer are fifty percent more likely to die than privately insured cancer patients.

Robert Wood Johnson Foundation. "Uninsured Americans with Chronic Health Conditions: Key Findings from the National Health Interview Survey." Cover the Uninsured Week 2005, May 2005. This report looks at the impact of chronic health conditions among the uninsured. Using data from the National

Center for Health Statistics' National Health Interview Survey (NHIS), the researchers found that: nearly half of all uninsured, non-elderly adults report having a chronic condition; many uninsured adults with chronic conditions do not have a usual source for health care; almost half of the uninsured adults with chronic conditions skip needed medical care or prescription drugs, because of cost; uninsured adults with chronic conditions skip needed medical care and prescription drugs at much higher rates than their do the insured; chronically ill uninsured adults are far less likely to visit a health professional than those with insurance; and uninsured adults with common chronic conditions suffer serious gaps in needed medical care.

Hadley, Jack and Peter J. Cunningham. "Issue Brief: Perception, Reality and Health Insurance: Uninsured as Likely as Insured to Perceive Need for Care but Half as Likely to Get Care." Center for Health System Change, October 2005. The insured and uninsured are just as likely to realize that they are in need of medical care; however, when they are sick, the insured will seek medical care eighty-two percent of the time, while the uninsured will only seek care thirty-seven percent of the time.

Kaiser Family Foundation. "The Uninsured: A Primer." The Kaiser Commission on Medicaid and the Uninsured, 2004. http://www.kff.org. This comprehensive report presents key facts about Americans without health insurance. Findings include: forty percent of the uninsured do not have a regular source of care, fifty percent delay seeking necessary care, and thirty-three percent say they did not receive necessary care. Twenty percent use a hospital's emergency room as a regular source of care. The uninsured are twice as likely as those with health insurance to live in a household that is having difficult paying monthly household expenses, and medical bills, and nearly twenty-five percent of the uninsured reported difficulty in paying medical bills. In addition, the uninsured sometimes pay higher hospital costs because they do not have the discounted rates that the privately insured have through the bargaining power of their insurance company.

Henry J. Kaiser Family Foundation. "Myths about the Uninsured." The Kaiser Commission on Medicaid and the Uninsured, April 28, 2005. This fact sheet discusses ten common myths about the uninsured. The majority of people who are uninsured do not choose to be uninsured; fifty-two percent of those without insurance say that cost is the main reason they lack health coverage for employer-based health insurance. The uninsured frequently go without needed care and are three times more likely to postpone needed care for major health conditions like injuries, pregnancy, and cancer than those with health coverage. This is in part because of the cost of care; most of the uninsured pay forty percent of their care directly, and many have real problems paying their medical bills.

Holes in the Safety Net

Kellermann, Arthur L. "Physician Support for Covering the Uninsured: Is the Cup Half Empty or Half Full?" Annals of Internal Medicine 139(10) (2003): 858–859. The uninsured are more likely to skip necessary and preventive care such as prenatal services than the insured. Therefore, the uninsured are more likely to die prematurely than the insured.

American College of Emergency Physicians. "EMTALA." 2006. This fact sheet gives an overview of the history and provisions of the Emergency Medical Treatment and Active Labor Act (EMTALA). Enacted in 1986, EMTALA is commonly referred to as the "anti-dumping law" because it requires all hospitals to provide a medical screening to all patients, even those without insurance, to ensure that they are stable enough for transfer to another hospital. After the enactment of EMTALA, hospitals became the only health care facility required by law to provide treatment to any individual, creating an essential safety net for those who need medical care but lack coverage. Hospitals and emergency physicians shoulder the financial burden of providing EMTALA-related care; each emergency physician on average provides $138,300 EMTALA-related charity care each year.

American College of Emergency Physicians. "The Uninsured: Access to Medical Care." June 2003. This fact sheet discusses the role of emergency rooms to meet the health care coverage needs of the uninsured. One out of three patients who come to hospital emergency rooms are uninsured, and twenty-five percent of them are children. According to this report, many of the uninsured who seek care in the emergency room are very sick because they have delayed needed care. Emergency rooms in hospitals are legally obligated to provide emergency care under a federal law (Emergency Medical Treatment and Act of Labor Act—EMTALA) that ensures that anyone who comes to an emergency room, regardless of their insurance status or ability to pay, must receive a medical screening exam and be stabilized. But many hospitals do not receive full payment for emergency services, and the authors estimate that fifty-five percent of all emergency care is uncompensated. Emergency physicians and other specialists combined lost $4.2 billion in revenue (2001) providing care under EMTALA. According to the American Medical Association, more than one-third of emergency physicians provide thirty hours of EMTALA-related care each week.

O'Malley, Ann S., Anneliese M. Gerland, Hoangmai H. Pham and Robert A. Berenson. "Issue Brief-Rising Pressure: Hospital Emergency Rooms as Barometers of the Health Care System." The Center for Health System Change, November 2005. This brief focuses on the challenges that emergency rooms face today, from persuading specialists to provide on-call coverage to treating the growing numbers of patients as more of the uninsured and underinsured come to emergency rooms for primary and specialty care. The authors note that hospitals today are under tremendous pressure to improve hospital system efficiency, directly conflicting with the increasing demands on hospital emergency rooms to provide more primary and uncompensated care for the uninsured.

Zigmond, Jessica. "No More Room: Overcrowding Blamed for Ambulance Diversions." Modern Health Care, February 13, 2006. According to a Centers for Disease Control Study, 16.2 million people arrived at emergency rooms for care in 2003, and of those sixteen-plus million, 501,000 were diverted to other hospitals because of a lack of appropriate beds in the emergency room. The number of emergency room visits rose by twenty-six percent from 1993 to 2003, while the number of emergency rooms decreased by twelve percent, leading to a state of serious overcrowding in our hospital emergency rooms. Ambulance diversion negatively affects the medical response system because the ambulance has to find another hospital thus increasing response time and travel time.

Alter, Harrison J. et al. "Health Status Disparities among Public and Private Emergency Department Patients." Academic Emergency Medicine 6(7) (1999): 736–743. This article examines the health and socioeconomic differences in patients who arrive in the emergency rooms of a public hospital versus a private hospital. Women and insured people were more likely to go to the private hospital, while African American and Latino patients were more likely to receive care in the public hospital. Patients who arrived at the public hospital were often sicker, in need of more urgent care, and had a higher rate of being uninsured. In general, patients who received care in the public hospital had significantly worse underlying health status than those who went to the private hospital.

Several newspaper stories cite statistics about emergency rooms and the uninsured:

Bill Smith, St. Louis Post-Dispatch, May 13, 2004. Lexis-Nexis. *"Many ER Patients Have No Insurance, Survey Finds/Another Key Finding: Most Are At or Over Capacity."* According to a national survey of 2000 emergency room physicians, one of every three patients who enters the emergency room is uninsured. Emergency rooms are experiencing overcrowding, with eighty-two percent of emergency rooms operating at or over capacity on weekdays, and ninety-one percent operating at or over capacity on weekends. The article also deals with the consequences of being uninsured: three-quarters of the physicians surveyed believed that the uninsured are more likely to die prematurely because of poorer health.

Libby, Leanne. *"Uninsured Treatment Is Hurting Hospitals: Cost in Texas Hit 6.7 Billion in 2002."* Corpus Christi Caller-Times. August 2, 2004. Lexis-Nexis. Treating the uninsured in emergency rooms limits access for everyone. This story discusses how one hospital in Corpus Christi, Texas, attempts to address unnecessary visits by referring uninsured patients with nonemergency problems to local clinics in the area for additional services. Texas spent $6.7 billion in charity care in 2002.

Song, Kyung M. *"ER Doctors Lament Rising Uninsured Load."* The Seattle Times. May 14, 2004. Lexis-Nexis. Emergency room physicians report that referrals to specialists, arranging follow-up treatments, and filling prescriptions are their toughest challenges in caring for uninsured patients. Manageable chronic illnesses such as diabetes or hypertension too often turn into major medical problems for patients without coverage, but disease management services to the uninsured are limited as an increasing number of private-practice physicians are refusing to accept both low-paying as well as uninsured patients. As a result, emergency rooms have become the usual source of care for increasing numbers of patients with non-emergency medical problems.

Whitney, David. *"Emergency Department Doctors Want Congressional Help."* McClatchy Newspapers, Washington Dateline. September 27, 2005. Lexis-Nexis. Emergency rooms suffer from the twin problems of treating larger numbers of the uninsured while finding it more difficult to find specialty physicians to provide on-call service. Hospitals are paying $600 million a year to ensure that on-call physicians are available, and still some communities cannot meet the need for specialty care in their hospital emergency rooms.

Going without Health Care Is Expensive Too

May, Jessica H. et al. "Issue Brief: Most Uninsured People Unaware of Health Care Safety Net Providers." Center for Health Systems Change, November 2004. The health care safety net includes those providers—physicians, clinics, and hospital emergency rooms—who offer free or reduced cost care to uninsured patients. Less than half of uninsured Americans use or are aware of safety net providers in their communities. Very few of the uninsured identify the hospital as a safety-net provider, despite the fact that visits to outpatient and emergency rooms make up more than half of all outpatient visits by uninsured people. This lack of awareness about available resources for health care may cause real problems for patients in rural areas that have limited safety net providers, since it will be important for the patients to know where the scarce resources are. The authors note that people who do not know about safety-net providers in their community will be more likely to skip necessary medical care.

A Nation's Health at Risk II: A Front Row Seat in a Changing Health Care System." National Association of Community Health Centers. August 2004. This report discusses the role of community health centers (CHCs) in providing health care to America's most vulnerable citizens. Forty percent of CHCs' patient population is uninsured, and the number of CHC patients continues to increase every year. According to the report, the number of people using ERs increased from 89.9 million in 1998 to 110.2 million in 2002, and increasing numbers of visits are for non-urgent reasons. The report suggests that CHCs provide significant savings for the health care system because they provide care and keep the uninsured from using emergency rooms (ERs) for non-emergency services. Redirecting non-urgent ER visits to more appropriate primary care settings would save more than $150 a visit. Since ten to fifty percent of ER visits are non-urgent, if the uninsured used CHCs instead of emergency rooms for primary care, between $1.6 billion to $8 billion in annual costs could be saved nationally.

CHAPTER 18

What Do We Spend Now?

Hadley, Jack and John Holahan. "The Cost of Care for the Uninsured: What Do We Spend, Who Pays, and What Would Full Coverage Add to Medical Spending: Issue Update." Kaiser Commission on Medicaid and the Uninsured, 2004. This 2004 report examines the cost of providing medical care to the uninsured, how much care the uninsured receive relative to fully insured people, and estimates the cost of additional medical care if the uninsured were provided and used health services at the rate of the insured population. Findings of the report include: 1) The uninsured used $125 billion in medical care in 2004; 2) The uninsured pay about thirty-five percent of their care as out-of-pocket expenditures (compared with twenty percent for the insured population), with government and private sources paying the rest; 3) Uncompensated care is estimated at $40.7 billion (2.7 percent of total personal health care in the U.S.); 4) The per-capita annual cost of medical care for the uninsured was $1,629 compared with $2,975 for the insured; 5) If the uninsured received full insurance coverage and utilized health services at the rate of their insured counterparts, total spending would increase by $48 billion (0.4-percent increase in Gross Domestic Product).

What Will It Cost?

Hadley, Jack and John Holahan. "Covering the Uninsured: How Much Would It Cost?" Health Affairs (June 4, 2003). This 2003 article suggests that the cost of additional medical care that would be used if the uninsured became insured would be less than generally thought. The authors make the following cost predictions based on public versus (higher) private reimbursement patterns, and suggest that an increase of $35 billion to $70 billion would provide health coverage to the uninsured. This would increase the health care portion of GDP less than one percentage point.

Families USA. "Paying a Premium: The Added Cost of Care for the Uninsured," June 2005. This report quantifies the dollar impact on private health insurance premiums to pay for health care provided to the uninsured. An estimated $43 billion in uncompensated care provided to the uninsured by hospitals and physicians are covered by three funding sources: private sources such as philanthropy; governmental programs that partially reimburse providers for the cost of care; and higher premiums for people with private health insurance. The authors estimate that the contribution of federal, state, and local public funds provide approximately one-third of the uncompensated care provided to the uninsured, and that the other two-thirds of the cost of uncompensated care is shifted to the private sector. As a result, premiums for family coverage include an extra $922 because of the cost of care for the uninsured, and individuals pay an extra $341—8.5% of each premium.

Dobson, Allen, Joan DaVanzo, and Namrata Sen. "The Cost-Shift Payment Hydraulic: Foundation, History, and Implications." Health Affairs 25(1) (2006): 22–33. The cost-shift payment is a fundamental aspect in American health care financing and places a burden on private payers to compensate for underfunded public programs and to help pay for uninsured patients. The article cites the Families USA study above (reference No. 4) that suggests that cost-shifting is a type of added "tax" on the premium, and that of the $40+ billion that is provided each year in uncompensated care, two-thirds ($29 billion) is "shifted" to the privately insured through higher family ($922) and individual ($341) insurance premiums.

Benner, Joshua A., Robert J. Glynn, Helen Mogun, Peter J. Neumann, Milton C. Weinstein, and Jerry Avorn. "Long-term Persistence in Use of Statin Therapy in Elderly Patients." JAMA 288(4) (2002): 455–461. This study showed that the use of statin therapy to reduce cholesterol decreased over time in older patients. The proportion of patients who took their statin therapy correctly was sixty percent after three months, forty-three percent after six months, and twenty-six percent after five years.

Jackevicius, Cynthia A., Muhammad Mamdani, Jack V. Tu. "Adherence With Statin Therapy in Elderly Patients with and without Acute Coronary Syndromes." JAMA 288(4) (2002): 462–467. The authors studied patients who had had: 1) severe chest pain or a heart attack in the last year; 2) those with evidence of chronic heart disease; and 3) those with no heart disease— all of whom had statins prescribed for high cholesterol. They found that, after two years of follow-up, only forty percent of patients in the chest pain/ heart attack group, thirty-six percent in the group with known heart disease, and twenty-five percent in the group with no known heart disease were still taking statins. Although those most healthy took statins the least, none of the groups took their medications as prescribed.

BlueCross BlueShield Association, "Medical Cost Reference Guide—4th Edition, 2006." This guide provides information on trends in the health care industry from national sources. The section entitled "National Healthcare Trends" lists private insurance administrative costs at fourteen percent.

Kaiser Permanente California. "Health Insurance Handbook." http://www .kaiserinsurancehealthcare.com (accessed April 2, 2006). This Kaiser Permanente Health plan web page reports that Kaiser Permanente has some of the lowest administrative costs in California; ninety-four percent is directed towards medical care, with only six percent for administration.

Weil, Alan. "There's Something about Medicaid." Health Affairs 22(1) (2003): 13–30. Medicaid is often used as an infrastructure for health coverage expansion efforts because of its flexibility and low administrative costs of less than five percent.

Newhouse, Joseph P. and Robert D. Reischauer. "The Institute of Medicine Committee's Clarion Call for Universal Coverage." Health Affairs 31 (March, 2004): W4-179-183. The authors of this article, two economists, suggest that expanding health insurance to the uninsured would be more costly than the IOM's estimate of $34 billion to $69 billion (2004 dollars) because any new program would also capture those who are currently underinsured who would also use more health services. The authors state that economic barriers against a national movement to expand health coverage are significant, even if introduced incrementally.

Miller, Wilhelmine, Elizabeth Richardson Vigdor, and Willard G. Manning. "Covering the Uninsured: What Is It Worth?" Health Affairs 31 (March, 2004): W4-157–167. Having one out of six working-age Americans without health insurance is costly to society in terms of increased mortality and poorer health. This article estimates the amount of "health capital" that someone loses or gains when they have stable health insurance coverage. Health capital is the value of income one can expect to receive over the course of one's life because one is healthy. It is estimated that the value of the "health capital" that would be gained as a result of insuring all Americans equals $65 billion to $130 billion per year for society as a whole.

Where Can We Find the Money?

Himmelstein, David and Steffie Woolhandler. "National Health Insurance or Incremental Reform: Aim High, or at Our Feet?" American Journal of Public Health. 93(1) (2003): 102–105. In this article the authors argue that single-payer national health insurance could cover the uninsured and upgrade coverage for most Americans without increasing costs, because savings on insurance overhead and other administrative costs would offset the costs of expanded coverage. According to the authors, if the U.S. reduced administrative spending in health care to Canadian levels we could save $140 billion annually.

Blendon, Robert J., John M. Benson and Catherine M. DesRoches. *"Americans' Views of the Uninsured: An Era for Hybrid Proposals." Health Affairs 27 (August 2003): W3-405-414.* Data from recent public opinion polls show that the cost of health care remains the most important health care issue in the minds of Americans. Many were not willing to pay more taxes to support such reforms. The authors suggest the major problem remains how to raise revenue to fund health insurance coverage for the uninsured.

Weisman, Jonathan. *"Congress Votes to Extend Tax Cuts." Washington Post 24 (September 2004), page A01.* This article discusses the Bush administration's first-term tax cut agenda worth nearly $1.9 trillion over ten years, and the late 2004 extension of three popular tax cuts worth $150 billion aimed at lower and middle-income tax payers.

Kamin, David and Isaac Shapiro. *"New Details Emerging on Effects of Recent Tax Cuts." Center of Budget and Policy Priorities, September 13, 2004.* This report analyzes the Bush administration tax cuts and cites, based on a Congressional Budget Office study, that the tax cuts will raise incomes (after taxes) by a much greater percentage for the top one percent of households than for any other income group. Those with the top one percent of household incomes will gain a 5.3 percent increase in after-tax income compared with a 1.5 percent gain for those with the lowest twenty percent of household income.

Kaiser Family Foundation. *Daily Health Policy Report, June 14, 2006, accessedhttp://www.kaisernetwork.org/daily_reports/rep_index.cfm?hint=3&DR_ID=37898.* The "Capitol Hill Watch" segment of this daily health policy report states that $94.5 billion in FY 2006 supplemental spending for the wars in Iraq and Afghanistan, border security, hurri-cane relief, and pandemic flu preparedness funds were approved by the House Appropriations Committee, with the Senate expected to concur.

CHAPTER 19

"What Does Canadian Citizenship Mean?" http://www.cic.gc.ca/english/ citizen/look. This government website says that Canadians value Equality, Cultural Differences, Freedom, Peace, and Law and Order. The phrase "peace, order, and good government," called POGG for short, is often used to describe the principles of the Canadian Confederation.

Mongan, James J. and Thomas H. Lee. *"Do We Really Want Broad Access to Health Care?"* New England Journal of Medicine 352(12) (2005): 1260–1263. This article points out the problems with the U.S. health care system and its lack of affordable, universal coverage. The authors cite examples of politics over policy during political campaigns, when promises and ideals regarding coverage, cost, and quality of health care don't get discussed or are forgotten after the election. Instead, elected officials continue funding safety net providers just enough to "move the care indoors and out of sight." The authors describe how Americans sacrifice in times of national crisis, but forget about their fellow Americans day in and day out, because they are "self-centered in the name of rugged individualism."

Appleby, Julie. *"Non-profit Hospitals' Top Salaries May Be Due for a Check-up."* USA TODAY September 29, 2004. http://usatoday.com/money/ industries/health/2004-19-29-nonprofit-salaries_x.htm. This article reports that hospital chief executive officers are among the top five highest-paid CEOs, regardless of for-profit or not-for-profit ownership status. In fact, CEOs at the six largest nonprofit hospitals make over $1.2 million a year. These salaries may have an impact on public views, particularly at a time when not-for-profit hospitals are being asked to demonstrate appropriate "community benefit" in exchange for their tax-exempt status.

Robinson, James C. *"Managed Consumerism in Health Care."* Health Affairs 24(6) (2005): 1478–1489. Two decades of experimentation with market-oriented health care reforms have failed to improve the health care system for America. This article suggests that the previous strategy of "managed competition" in which "regulated" health plans competed is being replaced by a more personal "consumer-directed" framework that focuses on individual behavior. The author believes that this generation of market-based strategies has promise because it focuses on individual choice, educated consumers, and competition, all of which could create an "efficient, fair and effective health care system." However, the author also cautions that if left unregulated, consumer-directed systems will penalize the sick and the poor as the healthy move out of insurance risk pools (leading to adverse selection) and the poor withholds necessary care because of the inability to pay for care.

Boaz, David. "Defining an Ownership Society." http://www.cato.org/cgi-bin/scripts/printtech.cgi/special/ownership_society/boaz.html. This article, from the Cato Institute, addresses calls for an "ownership society," and explores what that term means. The author believes that private ownership makes people more responsible and more involved. This type of philosophy extends into social programs in the form of school vouchers, private retirement accounts, and wider use of Health Savings Accounts in purchasing medical care.

Robinson, James C. "Health Savings Accounts—The Ownership Society in Health Care." New England Journal of Medicine 353(12) (2005): 1199–1202. In this article, the author explores the use of health savings accounts (HSAs) as an example of the president's "ownership agenda." According to the author, HSAs fit the American philosophy of "less government" and a belief in privatization. This type of health care financing vehicle shifts paying for health care from an insurance model to a savings model and will serve some Americans better than others, generally the healthier and wealthier, who will benefit from the tax-advantaged health savings accounts and who may not have a need for comprehensive health insurance.

The Economist. "Desperate Measures." Special Report: America's Health-care Crisis, 28 February 2006. This article examines whether market-based health care reforms, such as HSAs, will be effective in expanding coverage to uninsured Americans. The authors note that the shift to consumer-directed health care with its greater sharing of cost with the consumer will involve a culture change from the traditional employer-based health care model and may take years to complete. As the young and healthy leave traditional risk-sharing insurance pools for HSAs, the poor and sick who depend upon comprehensive coverage will be left unable to afford the rising insurance premiums. The article concludes with a prediction that the current health agenda may speed certain incremental reforms like greater cost consciousness only to weaken the overall system in the long run by segregating the sick from the well, which undermines any sense of a "social contract" between the government and its most vulnerable citizens.

Schudson, Michael. "The News Media as Political Institutions." *Annual Review of Political Science* 5(2002): 249–269. Investigators in sociology, communications, and political science have studied the role of the media from different perspectives. This review article discusses the different views surrounding the cultural influences of the media and its role in shaping public opinion and in influencing belief systems, assumptions, and values. The article mentions that for many scholars, and most lay people, the model of media influence is a "hypodermic" model in which the media injects ideas into a passive public. The author prefers to think of the media as a cultural producer and messenger of cultural meanings and symbols, which provides to consumers a "web" of meanings that relate to how people live their lives.

Otten, Alan L. "The Influence of the Mass Media on Health Policy." *Health Affairs* (Winter 1992): 111–118. The author notes that television and "sound bites" will continue to be the way most Americans receive information and opinion, but that there are also quality TV news shows that compensate for the typical "sound-bite journalism."

Annas, George J. "Reframing the Debate on Health Care Reform by Replacing Our Metaphors." *New England Journal of Medicine* 332(11) (1995): 745–748. In this article, the author examines how the U.S. uses market comparisons to describe health care: "portraying efficiency, profit maximization, customer satisfaction, the ability to pay, planning, and competitive models," which reflected the "corporatization" of medicine of the 1990s. The author suggests that the health care "language" in politics and policy must move toward an "ecological" metaphor of "conservation and sustainability."

Mechanic, David. "Muddling Through Elegantly: Finding the Proper Balance in Rationing." *Health Affairs* 16(5) (1997): 83–92. The article explores the tensions between the promise of (and demand for) medical advances and the need for controlling cost in the U.S. health care system. The author argues that the American public will resist rationing and "wants it all."

Truog, Robert D. et al. "Rationing in the Intensive Care Unit." *Critical Care Medicine*. 34(4) (2006): 958–963. Efforts to ration care in intensive care units (ICUs) have failed because many patients and families believe they are entitled to any available service (regardless of its benefit), and many clinicians believe they must, in the name of professional duty to the patient, offer any service that yields even minimal benefit. This article offers possible guidelines in developing a system to ration care reasonably in a critical-care setting.

Blendon, Robert J. et al. "Voters and Health Care in the 2004 Election." Health Affairs 1 (March 2005): 447–457. Exit polls after the 2004 presidential race showed that health care did not matter much as an election issue. This article breaks down how Americans voted in the 2004 and suggests that moral values, jobs and the economy, and terrorism all were more important to voters than health care. Health care issues were most important with women, the elderly, African Americans, and low-income voters. The authors suggest that the greatest policy challenge within health reform efforts will be to try for consensus on policy priorities and policy solutions.

Bodenheimer, Thomas. "The Political Divide in Health Care: A Liberal Perspective." Health Affairs 24(6) (2005): 1426–1447. U.S. health policy rests between conservative and liberal viewpoints, which basically part along lines of whether health care coverage is a basic right or not. This article lobbies for a return to a more liberal perspective where the concerns of an entire population are more important than the individual, and an insurance model is created that provides universal coverage, equitable financing of health care, and a commitment to equality in health care services.

Pear, Robert. "Medicare Law Prompts a Rush for Lobbyists." New York Times, August 23, 2005. This article reports that the amount spent on federal lobbying for health care equaled $325 million in 2004, more than any other sector. Within that amount, drug companies led spending with $86.9 million, hospitals spent $55 million, and physician groups spent $35.4 million on federal lobbying activities.

American Enterprise Institute. "New AEI Public Opinion Study on Taxes." April 13, 2006. This press release issued just before tax day on April 15 reported on surveys by major U.S. pollsters on the topic of taxes. Findings include: most Americans say the amount of taxes they pay is too high; only one in ten Americans would be willing to pay the extra $2,470 per person in taxes to balance the federal budget deficit and six in ten believe that if they paid the extra taxes the government would simply increase spending rather than balance the budget; and eighty-six percent of Americans favor elimination of the estate tax.

Oberlander, Jonathan. "The Politics of Health Reform: Why Do Bad Things Happen to Good Plans?" Health Affairs 27 (August 2003): 433–446.

The author discusses the various unsuccessful attempts at comprehensive health reform over the last fifty years, and suggests that one reason for the lack of major reform is that incremental changes are more attractive to most Americans, notably in the form of either tax credits or expansion of public programs. However, experience with incremental "fixes" in the past such as HIPAA or SCHIP have not brought long-term success in alleviating the access or cost problems in the U.S. health care system, and often end up mostly maintaining the status quo. Despite the fact that many citizens and elected officials say that we can no longer sustain the status quo in American health care, the author notes that, based on historical precedent, the status quo almost always becomes the preferred choice as soon as comprehensive health reform makes it onto the political agenda.

Steinmo, Sven and Jon Watts. "Why Comprehensive National Health Insurance Always Fails in America." *Journal of Health Politics, Policy and Law 20(2) (1995).* This article discusses why national health reform is so difficult to achieve in the United States because of a bias against comprehensive reform. Reasons for the failure to enact a national program were the same in 1994 (the last attempt) as they were in 1948, 1965, 1974, and 1978. They include the role of interest groups, a weak executive branch, a fragmented political party system, an American distaste for a large government, and a system of checks and balances. As a result, incremental reforms are more possible and more popular.

Machiavelli, Niccolo. *The Prince,* accessed at: http://www.quotationspage .com/quote/20613.html.

CHAPTER 20

Previous Plans Failed Because They Forgot Who We Are

Zelman, Walter and Lawrence D. Brown. "Looking Back on Health Care Reform: 'No Easy Choices'." *Health Affairs 17(6) (1998): 61–68.* This almost decade-old article represents a discussion from one of the Clinton Health Plan architects (Walter Zelman) about why the proposed national plan failed, and what we can learn from it. Interest group attacks, the secrecy of how the plan was put together, and the complexity of the plan all led toward its defeat, despite the fact that its design attempted to blend government regulation and market forces. The authors note that American political institutions and the American philosophy of limited government all point toward incremental, rather than wide-ranging, reforms.

Skocpol, Theda. *Boomerang: Health Care Reform and the Turn Against Government*. W. W. Norton and Company: New York/London 1997, 240 pages. In this book, Skocpol describes what she perceives as several major reasons for the failure of the Clinton health reform plan and the subsequent conservative revolt. Some of the reasons include: the number and complexity of issues requiring the balance between market-oriented and government-centered reform ideas ended up angering those it hoped to satisfy; the disorganized and delayed reform plan was killed by a united attack (involving the insurance industry among others) which had more credibility with American citizens; and the anti-tax, anti-government legacy of President Reagan that was played out as a "mobilization against government." As a result, politicians interpreted the failure of the health reform bill as a national directive to limit health policy initiatives to incremental expansions. The author suggests that unregulated competition and tax cuts for the wealthy (without real change in government programs) cannot produce medical care security for the sixty percent of Americans at the lower end of the income scale; these people could provide the momentum for another attempt at health care reform.

West, Darrell M. Diane Health, and Chris Goodwin. "Harry and Louise Go to Washington: Political Advertising and Health Care Reform." *Journal of Health Politics, Policy and Law* 21(1) (1996): 35 68. This article dis cusses the role and impact that the media and political advertising had in influencing public opinion in 1993 and 1994 during President Clinton's health reform initiative. Over 650 interest groups spent $60 million on lobbying for and against the reform plan. The health insurance industry led one of the more successful advertising campaigns with the "Harry and Louise" commercials, which were geared toward the "average American." These ads were particularly successful because most Americans did not understand the plan, and therefore were influenced by the commercials against the proposed program. According to the authors of this paper, there was little to no restraint in the media during this time, as news accounts during the health plan debate focused on the sensational, amplified claims of special interests, thus swaying public opinion.

Steinmo, Sven and Jon Watts. "Why Comprehensive National Health Insurance Always Fails in America." Journal of Health Politics, Policy and Law 20(2) (1995). This article discusses why national health reform is so difficult to achieve in the United States because of a bias against comprehensive reform of the system. Reasons for the failure to enact a national program were the same in 1994 (the last attempt) as they were in 1948, 1965, 1974, and 1978, and include: the role of interest groups, a weak executive branch, a fragmented political party system, American distaste for large government, and a system of "checks and balances" that makes consensus by large numbers of individuals and groups required to move any new legislation forward. As a result, incremental reforms are more feasible and more popular.

Gilmer, Todd and Richard Kronick. "It's the Premiums, Stupid: Projections of the Uninsured through 2013." Health Affairs April 5, 2005: W5-143-151. According to the authors, the number of uninsured will grow to fifty-six million by 2013; for each one-percent increase in health spending over personal income, 246,000 people will lose private health insurance coverage.

Schoen, Cathy, Michelle M. Doty, Sara R. Collins, and Alyssa L. Holmgren. "Insured but Not Protected: How Many Adults Are Underinsured?" Health Affairs 2005 Web Exclusive June 14, 2005; W5-289-302. This study uses financial risk to define what is meant by the term "underinsured" with three criteria: (1) medical expenses amounted to ten percent of income or more; (2) among low-income adults (below 200 percent FPL), medical expenses amounted to at least five percent of income; and (3) health plan deductibles equaled or exceeded five percent of income. When assessing the results of a national health insurance survey, the authors found that three of four people aged nineteen to sixty-four said that they had been insured all year, and when the three indicators of uninsurance were applied, twelve percent of the insured adults—nearly sixteen million—were underinsured. When uninsured adults (forty-six million) were added to those who were underinsured based on financial indicators, an estimated sixty-one million adults, or thirty-five percent of the population aged nineteen to sixty-four, had either no insurance, some coverage, or insurance that exposed them to "catastrophic" medical costs during 2003.

Bad and Getting Worse

Agency for Health Care Research and Quality. "One Quarter of Nonelderly Poor in the United States without Health Insurance from 2000–2003." www.meps.aharq.gov/papers/st123/stat123.pdf. In a 2006 report looking at the long-term uninsured in the U.S., the Agency for Healthcare Research and Quality (ARHQ) reports that 24.2 percent of poor Americans under the age of sixty-five—3.8 million persons—reported being continuously uninsured through either private or public insurance for at least four years when surveyed in 2003.

Concepts and Goals for Reform

Davis, Karen. "Aiming High: Targets for the U.S. Health System." The Commonwealth Fund. 2005. http://www.cmwf.org. Part of the 2005 Annual Report from the Commonwealth Fund, this message from president Karen Davis identifies ten core values around which the U.S. health care system should be organized, and then defines actions to address some of the current problems. Examples of some of the core values include living "long, healthy, and productive lives, receiving the right care," and "receiving efficient high-value care." Citing a study of the National Committee for Quality Assurance, the U.S. would reduce mortality rates by approximately 50,000 deaths per year at a cost savings of $3.5 billion if all health plans provided the same level of quality care as the best performing plans. To tackle some of the problems in our health care system, the author recommends rewarding more efficient and high quality medical care providers, improving patient care management, expanding the use of information technology, and using practice guidelines based upon evidence.

Zuckerman, Stephan and Joshua McFeeters. "Recent Growth in Health Expenditures." The Commonwealth Fund. March 2006. Health care expenditures have continued to grow faster than the Gross Domestic Product (GDP). This article discusses trends in health care spending and blames a large part of our increased spending on new technology and increased use of medical care. Large administrative expenses (thirty percent) and increasing prices have all contributed to the growth in health expenditures.

The authors suggest that new approaches, such as consumer-directed strategies, pay-for-performance, and chronic disease management, will be considered alongside the more traditional strategies of government price-setting in future attempts to reduce the rate of growth in health expenditures. Without cost controls, health care expenditures could reach twenty percent of GDP by 2015.

An Approach to Change

Garson, Arthur Jr. "Health Care for All of U.S: Start with the States." Harvard Health Policy Review 5(1) (2004): 47–54. U.S. health care reform is not likely to emerge as a major national issue unless and until the eighty-five percent of Americans with health coverage express dissatisfaction and bring political pressure to elected officials. Because of this lack of national attention, there may be opportunities for states to implement innovative health programs at the state level. This article discusses some possible state models to improve affordable health coverage and cites as examples the Healthy New York and Maine Dirigo Health Programs. The author suggests electronic claims processing, reduction of wasteful overuse of health services, and a dedicated tax on fast food as ways to increase funding.

Harvard Interfaculty Program for Health Systems Improvement. "A Strategy for Health Care Reform: Catalyzing Change from the Bottom Up." Cambridge: Harvard University Press, 2006. This study makes a number of recommendations for incremental change including state reforms and then recommends eventual comprehensive change.

Davis K., A. Garson, and the Committee on Rapid Advances Demonstration Projects: Health Care Finance and Delivery Systems. State Health Insurance: Making Affordable Coverage Available to All Americans. Institute of Medicine; Washington, DC, National Academies Press (2002) pages 69–76. This study makes recommendations for health care reform using state demonstration projects to extend coverage and control costs.

Garson, Arthur. "U.S. Health Care: The Intertwined Caduceus of Physicians, Coverage, Quality and Cost." Journal of American College of Cardiology 43(1) (2004): 1–5. Physicians can take a leadership role in improving the health care system, both by improving individual patient care and by improving the systems through which medical care is delivered. The author suggests that promoting a coordinated approach to care through state-level demonstrations and by linking payments to the adoption of evidence-based practices will improve health coverage, patient safety, and quality of care. The author notes that reducing administrative costs from eight percent to four percent would save $60 billion per year.

Thorpe, Kenneth. "Impacts of Health Care Reform: Projections of Costs and Savings." National Coalition on Health Care, 2005. This report by the National Coalition on Health Care sets out objectives for health care reform and the potential costs and savings of four scenarios. In all four scenarios, the authors found that the cost of a reformed system would be less than the cost of continuing the way we are. The authors report that forty percent of today's eighteen billion health care transactions are still done in paper form and that moving to electronic billing, claims processing, and payment would save $30 billion in administrative costs.

Gauthier, Anne, Stephen C. Schoenbaum, and Ilana Weinbaum. "Toward a High Performance Health System for the United States." The Commonwealth Fund. March 2006. http://www.cmwf.org. This report examines how the U.S. health care system falls short on performance as a result of fragmented organizational and payment systems. The authors note that public and private payers can promote reform through investments in research and through improvements in efficiency. Rather than comprehensive transformation of the U.S. health care system, these authors suggest that a more politically feasible, incremental redesign of the basic private-public system could yield significant improvements in health care coverage, cost, and quality.

Fronstin, Paul. "Workers' Health Insurance: Trends, Issues, and Options to Expand Coverage." The Commonwealth Fund. March 2006. http://www.cmwf.org. In recent years, employer-sponsored health insurance has been decreasing, particularly in small businesses, causing an associated decrease in the number of working adults with health insurance coverage. Currently, only fifty-nine percent of small employers offered health insurance in 2005, down from sixty-three percent in 2004. This article discusses reasons for this trend and examines private and public approaches to expand health coverage for workers, including tax credits, Association Health Plans, state high-risk pools, and reinsurance.

Collins, Sara R., K. Davis, M. M. Doty, J. L. Kriss, and A. L. Holmgren. "Gaps in Health Insurance: An All-American Problem." The Commonwealth

Fund, April 2006. Findings from the Commonwealth Fund Biennial Health Insurance Survey show that lack of insurance is highest among families with incomes under $20,000 (fifty-three percent). This is similar to past surveys, but these findings also suggest that uninsurance rates for moderate- and middle-income earners ($20,000–$40,000) and their families increased to forty-one percent in 2005, up from twenty-eight percent in 2001.

Attempts to Improve Options for Small Business

Employee Benefit Research Institute. "Has There Been a Shift to Small Firms? The Impact of Firm Size on Employment-Based Health Benefits." EBRI Notes, accessed at www.ebri.org, Volume 25(8) (2004), 3. This article examines changes in the distribution health insurance among different size firms. Firms with fewer than 500 employees account for much of the new job growth in the U.S., yet workers in small firms are much less likely to have health benefits than workers in large firms. In 2004, 60.5 percent of uninsured Americans were in families whose family head was employed in a firm with fewer than 500 employees.

Enthoven, Alain. "Employment-based Health Insurance Is Failing: Now What?" Health Affairs (2003): W3-237-249. The author states that employer-based health insurance is failing because costs are out of control. He argues that it is in the best interest of employers and employees to move to a system that offers a range of choices in health plans and that reflects both employees' preferences and ability to pay. He advocates for a "managed competition" model with insurance "exchanges" that rely on fixed contributions from employers and are portable from job to job. This was the basis for the "Health Security Act" proposed by the Clinton administration. Employees would choose plans and pay the difference in premiums depending upon their health care preferences and their willingness and ability to pay. The author believes that people would be cost-conscious, and claims that this type of system would have the advantage of freeing employers from the burden of purchasing health benefits for their employees, would reduce administrative costs, and would allow choice. This, in turn, would ultimately decrease cost and improve quality as regulated insurance companies competed for enrollees. He cites the Federal Employees Health Benefits Plan (FEHBP) as an example of a successful managed competition model.

"Insurance Markets: What Health Insurance Pools Can and Can't Do."
California Health Care Foundation. November 2005. Health insurance purchasing pools may be attractive models to lower the cost of purchasing
health insurance for small businesses and individuals, although they also
have their limitations. This study suggests that insurance pools do not in fact
lower premiums nor decrease the number of uninsured. There are two
main reasons why pools do not work: 1) Larger group plans have economies
of scale that yield lower administrative costs, whereas small employers and
the self-employed have the choice to leave a pooled arrangement if the cost
of health coverage becomes too expensive. This may cause insurance pools
to have adverse selection because the small businesses that choose to remain in the pools may have sicker employees who need health coverage; 2)
Unless a pool can attract and maintain a large number of enrollees, it will
not have economies of scale nor be able to negotiate with health plans.

*EP&P Consulting, Inc. Healthy New York: Executive Summary, Decem-
ber 31, 2005.* This executive summary reviews the "Healthy New York"
(Healthy NY) program and its successes. Healthy NY was developed in January of 2001 as a public/private insurance program that offers health insurance benefits to small companies, the self-employed, and workers who cannot obtain insurance from an employer. The program has twenty-one health
plans, all of which use a "stop-loss reinsurance" fund that pays for all claims
over $30,000 and therefore decreases risk and keeps premiums below mar-
ket rate. As of December 2005, there were 106,944 active enrollees in the
Healthy NY program. In general, enrollees and health plans reported satisfaction with Healthy NY. Despite the fact that thirty-eight percent of the
people below 200 percent of the Federal Poverty Level in New York still
lack health coverage, Healthy NY is considered a state-wide success and
looked upon as a winning strategy to provide affordable insurance coverage
for those least likely to obtain insurance.

*Swartz, Katherine. "Healthy New York: Making Insurance More Afford-
able for Low-Income Workers." The Commonwealth Fund. November
2001.* This briefing summarizes the Healthy New York health insurance
purchasing alliance program and suggests improvements to further expand
enrollment. Of the 8.2 million working adults in New York State, twenty-
five percent worked in businesses that did not offer health insurance.
Healthy NY offers a health insurance program with premiums that are
thirty to fifty percent lower than the individual market ($200 compared

with $340), with similar reductions in the small-group market rates, and is available to low-income workers in small businesses and to low-income adults who lack access to employer-sponsored coverage. The program has reduced benefits and a restricted network of providers, and relies on the state to provide a ninety percent re-insurance benefit for large medical expenses between $30,000 and $100,000; after that point the insurer provides the reinsurance. The authors suggest that enrollment could be expanded by providing direct premium subsidies to individuals to purchase coverage and by broadening the choice of benefits.

Academy Health. "State of the States." State Coverage Initiatives, 2006 edition. This annual report updates enrollment and program features of the Healthy NY program, a state-subsidized health insurance program. In 2005, Healthy NY had 100,000 enrollees, and averaged more than 7,000 new enrollees per month in 2005. Approximately fifty-seven percent are working individuals employed by companies that do not offer health insurance, eighteen percent are individuals who own their own businesses, and twenty-five percent are enrolled through small business groups.

Office of Personnel Management. "Federal Employees Health Benefits Program." http://www.opm.gov/insure/health/about/fehb.asp. The Federal Employee Health Benefit Program (FEHBP) provides federal employees with a variety of health plan choices, ranging from traditional fee-for-service to less expensive but more restricted Health Maintenance Organizations. On average, the federal government pays seventy-two percent of the insurance premium and never more than seventy-five percent of the premium. The program provides enrollees with comparisons of benefits and costs by mail and e-mail.

Davis, Karen, Barbara Cooper, and Rose Capasso. "The Federal Employee Health Benefits Program: A Model for Workers, Not Medicare." The Commonwealth Fund. November 2003. This brief describes the Federal Employee Health Benefits Program (FEHBP) for 8.5 million federal employees. It uses a "managed competition" model to encourage beneficiaries to make cost-conscious decisions through the provision of a defined contribution (a fixed payment) for health insurance premiums that can be applied toward many different insurance products. This provides economies of scale to keep the administrative costs low and encourages members to choose plans that are less expensive. The authors suggest that the FEHBP model could provide a pool that could work within the individual and small business insurance markets.

Norris, Kim. "Sharing Health Coverage: Three-Pronged Medical Care." Detroit Free Press. October 25, 2004. http://www.freep.com. Health Choice is a so-called "three-share" program in which employers, workers, and the government share in the cost of health care. Started in 1994 in Wayne County, Michigan, low-income small businesses with more than three workers are eligible to participate in the program. Workers who make $10 an hour or less are eligible for the full one-third government-share subsidy, while workers who make more receive less. At one point, Health Choice enrolled more than 20,000 people, but failure to pay providers in a timely manner led many physicians to discontinue seeing Health Choice enrollees, and membership fell to 5,000. The county restructured the program in 2004 and 2005 and set fees at $170 per month split three ways ($57 each). Despite its troubles, the program has been successful in containing costs and improving health outcomes as it expands coverage to the low-income working uninsured.

"Michigan: Access Health." The Commonwealth Fund, October 2004; Muskegon Community Health Project, http://www.mchp.org/index.html. Access Health, developed by Muskegon Community Health Project (MCHP), is an innovative approach to provide health coverage to uninsured working families in Muskegon County, Michigan. Over 400 local small businesses and 1,500 people annually participate in the program. It is built upon a three-share model that distributes the cost among employer, employee, and the community, allowing small- and mid-sized businesses to provide a benefit plan that includes local physician services, in-patient hospitalization, out-patient services, emergency services, behavioral health, prescription drugs, diagnostic lab and x-rays, home health, and hospice care. Access Health provides county subsidies (funded by Medicaid dollars) to employers and employees of low-income, small firms. In 2003, Access Health covered 1,500 workers and 400 businesses. The employer and employee each pay thirty percent of the premium, and the county pays forty percent.

French, Rose. "Bredesen Signs Cover Tennessee." The Tennessean, June 13, 2006. This Associated Press news item reports that the governor of Tennessee, Governor Bredesen, signed into law the new health care program called Cover Tennessee, which will provide subsidized health insurance for low-income workers, and in which the premium costs will be shared among employers, employees, and the state. The state estimates that 190,000 residents will enroll over the next three years.

Davis, Karen, Michelle M. Doty and Alice Ho. "How High Is Too High? Implications of High-Deductible Health Plans." The Commonwealth Fund. April 2005: iii-viii. This study examines the use of high deductible health plans (HDHP). HDHPs claim to lower health care costs by causing patients to be more cost conscious and by making insurance premiums more affordable for the uninsured. However, the authors found that HDHPs are not likely to have a positive effect on either costs or coverage, and may defeat the basic purpose of health insurance, because largely healthy people sign up for them and there is less money available to spread the risk of high-cost patients. In their view, HDHPs do not work well for low-income populations (below 200 percent Federal Poverty Level) or for those who have chronic health problems. For these groups, insurance premiums can range from six to twenty percent of income, and out-of-pocket expenses can exceed twenty-six percent of income. Unless HDHPs provide lower deductibles for low-income or chronically ill patients, these types of plans may keep such patients from seeking medical care.

Glied, Sherry et al. "Barebones Health Plans: Are They Worth the Money?" Issue Brief No. 518, The Commonwealth Fund, May 2002. Health insurance premiums rise with the benefits included in the plan: the more generous the health plan, the more expensive. This study examines "bare bones" insurance policies and asks whether the cost reductions reduce access to needed health care services. The most common way to increase affordability of health insurance is to increase the share of expenses that patients must pay out of pocket, such as for deductibles, co-insurance, and co-payments. Without changing the benefits in a plan, to achieve a thirty-percent savings in premium would require a very large increase in deductible, for example to $1,300. The author argues that because the average uninsured individual has an annual income of $11,883, it is questionable whether a "reduced" health insurance premium of $1,450 with a deductible of $1,300 will work. The combination of the premium and deductible would easily exceed ten percent of income, a percentage that is unrealistic relative to other household needs for low-wage workers.

Attempts to Improve the Safety Net

Achman, Lori and Deborah Chollet. "Insuring the Uninsurable: An Overview of State High-Risk Pools." The Commonwealth Fund, August 2001. The report analyzes the use and success of state high-risk insurance pools. The authors find that high-risk pools do provide an alternative for individuals who have no employer-sponsored health insurance but do have extensive health care needs and medical expenses, but that average individual premiums are high ($5,000) and often include restrictions on benefits like mental health and maternity. Although some states (Minnesota) insure up to six percent of their individually insured population through high risk pools, that is unusual; most states insure less than one percent.

Council for Affordable Health Insurance. "2005 State Legislators' Guide to Health Insurance Solutions," www.alec.org. This guide to health insurance solutions at the state level presents various options for states to explore in trying to expand health coverage and control health costs. It reports that state high-risk pools are one way to provide comprehensive health insurance to those who are medically uninsurable because of health risk, that these types of pools have been around for twenty-five years, and that in 2004, 172,000 people in thirty-four states were covered under high-risk pools.

Collins, Sara R. et al. "Wages, Health Benefits, and Workers' Health." The Commonwealth Fund, publication No. 788, October 2004. This study finds major coverage differences between higher-wage earners and low-wage earners, with higher-wage earners being more likely to have insurance and health-related benefits. Despite these differences, the authors conclude that because of the strong public support for employer-based coverage and a growing federal deficit making it unlikely to expand public programs, any health care reform will likely have to build on the employer-based insurance structure.

Hadley, Jack and Timothy Waidman. "Health Insurance and Health at Age 65: Implications for Medical Care Spending on New Medicare Beneficiaries." Health Services Research 41(2) (2006): 429–451. This study examines the impact of lowering the age of Medicare enrollment to age fifty-five with regard to health status and long-term costs to the public program. The authors report that extending insurance to all Americans between the ages of fifty-five and sixty-four would improve health and increase survival, and at age sixty-five, could reduce short-term spending by Medicare for newly eligible enrollees, even though more people would enter the program.

Eddy, David M. "Health System Reform: Will Controlling Costs Require Rationing of Services?" JAMA 272(4) (1994): 324–328. This article discusses the growth of medical spending and the reasons why medical spending has outpaced the growth in GDP by three percent for over thirty years. The author suggests that neither administrative efficiencies nor elimination of waste in the health care system will be enough to permanently control health spending because the demand for services and the price of services will continue to grow each year, because of the demand for and availability of technology, the aging of the population, and the continual discovery of new ways to prevent some diseases and diagnose and treat others. Ultimately, according to the author, we will have to make decisions about how to ration our resources if we are serious about cost control.

Where Do We Go from Here?

Near-Term: Incremental Change

Collins, Sara R., Karen Davis and Alice Ho. "Opinion: Proposals for Health Policy. A Shared Responsibility: U.S. Employers and the Provision of Health Insurance to Employees." Inquiry 42 (2005): 6–15. This article examines the characteristics of employer-based health insurance and discusses the advantages, including benefits to employers and the presence of better benefits to workers and administrative efficiencies. The article also discusses the steady reduction in percentage of workers covered even by large employers and the need to strengthen how employer coverage works because of reports that suggest that even in large companies health coverage is increasingly difficult to obtain because of complex administrative rules. However, rather than dismantle the existing system, the authors suggest policies such as tax credits and other premium supports that might strengthen and expand employer coverage.

Reschovsky, James D. "Employer Health Insurance Premium Subsidies Unlikely to Enhance Coverage Significantly." Issue Brief. Center for Studying Health System Change. No. 46, December 2001. State and local efforts to reduce the number of uninsured workers include three major approaches: public insurance expansions, subsidies to employees to purchase employer-sponsored health insurance or insurance in the individual market, or subsidies paid directly to small employers to make offering health insurance more affordable. Low-wage, uninsured workers in small firms would need a large subsidy to use offered health insurance coverage; it is estimated that a subsidy of thirty percent would only yield a three-percent decrease in the number of uninsured. The authors discuss the difficulties in providing incentives to purchase insurance through subsidies, either at the individual or the small business level, mainly because in order to be effective, the size of the subsidy would have to be quite large and therefore costly.

Cogan, John F., R. Glenn Hubbard and Daniel P. Kessler. "Making Markets Work: Five Steps to a Better Health Care System." Health Affairs 24(6) (2005): 1447–1457. In response to the article above, this article takes the conservative view and argues that market forces should dictate the answer to a health care system marked by waste. The authors suggest tax reforms (full deductibility of insurance premiums for individuals and tax credits), insurance reforms (health savings accounts), improved availability of information, enhanced competition (federal regulations for insurance), subsidies for the chronically ill, and malpractice reforms as required principles for a system that relies on choice and value.

Aaron, Henry J. and Stuart M. Butler. "How Federalism Could Spur Bipartisan Action on the Uninsured." Health Affairs Web Exclusive (March 31, 2004): W4-168-178. National efforts to reduce the numbers of Americans without health insurance have made little progress over the decades because achieving majority support for any one approach on a nationwide basis has been impossible. The authors suggest that federally supported state experimentation would be a promising way to make progress, and that states should be allowed to try different approaches with funding linked to success in reaching identified expanded health coverage goals within state.

Long, Sharon K., Stephen Zuckerman, and John A. Graves. "Are Adults Benefiting from State Coverage Expansions?" Health Affairs 17 (January 2005): W1-14. This study provides an evaluation of state efforts to expand insurance coverage by providing health insurance to parents whose children qualified for existing state programs. Looking at expansion programs in California, Wisconsin, New Jersey, and Massachusetts, the study found that insurance coverage did increase with public expansion programs; in Massachusetts and Wisconsin, people stayed with their private insurance, thus resulting in a net gain in the number of uninsured, whereas in California and New Jersey, most who went into the public system had been previously covered by private insurance, with little overall gain.

S. 2772, *introduced in U.S. Senate May 9, 2006. Accessed at: http:// thomas.loc.gov/cgi-bin/thomas.* A bill to provide for innovation in health care through state initiatives that expand coverage and access and improve quality and efficiency in the health care system; to the Committee on Health, Education, Labor, and Pensions.

Altman, Stuart and Michael Doonan. "Can Massachusetts Lead the Way in Health Care Reform?" New England Journal of Medicine 354(20) (2006): 2093–2095. Massachusetts passed legislation in the spring of 2006 that calls for universal insurance coverage for its citizens beginning in 2007. The plan includes an individual mandate to have health insurance, expands public insurance programs to include everyone under 100 percent of the Federal Poverty Level, and provides new health insurance options and pooling for the low-income and for small businesses.

Himmelstein, David and Steffie Woolhandler. "National Health Insurance or Incremental Reform: Aim High, or at Our Feet?" American Journal of Public Health. 93(1) (2003): 102–105. In this article the authors argue that single-payer national health insurance could cover the uninsured and upgrade coverage for most Americans without appreciatively increasing costs if we were able to capture the thirty percent of health dollars that currently fund administration, overhead, and profits within our current private/public system. They admit that incremental reform is more politically feasible, but they claim that little will get accomplished with small changes.

Deber, Raisa Berlin. "Health Care Reform: Lessons from Canada." American Journal of Public Health 93(1) (2003): 20–24. Although there are many criticisms about the Canadian health care system, access, quality, and satisfaction are relatively high in Canada, and spending is relatively well controlled. This article describes the structure of Canadian health care and the current challenges facing the system, mostly having to do with financing. Lessons for the U.S. include the importance of providing all citizens with access to basic health care, the administrative efficiencies within a single-payer system, and the fact that regional systems can operate within a larger national structure.

Fuchs, Victor R. and Ezekiel J. Emanuel. "Health Care Reform: Why? What? When?" Health Affairs 24(6) (2005): 1399–1413. Although dissatisfaction within the U.S. health care system is widespread and long-standing, no consensus has emerged regarding reform. The authors of this article discuss types of incremental and comprehensive reform strategies, and suggest that incremental reform is more politically feasible in the U.S., but not as effective in reducing costs and increasing coverage as comprehensive reform. The authors discuss the challenges that comprehensive reformers face when trying to make large reforms at the national level, and argue that major reform is likely to come in response to major social upheaval, such as a war, an economic downturn, or large-scale civil unrest.

Oberlander, Jonathan. "The Politics of Health Reform: Why Do Bad Things Happen to Good Plans?" Health Affairs 27 (August 2003): 433–446. Just because comprehensive health reform is politically desirable may not make it feasible, the author contends in this article, and suggests that feasibility is why incremental reforms are proposed. In his view, the three most overlooked lessons from U.S. health policies are: 1) getting reform on the national agenda does not mean it will pass; 2) consensus that a problem exists implies no agreement on solutions; and 3) favorable public opinion does not guarantee legislative victory. Therefore, designing comprehensive health reform plans is unlikely to overcome these problems, because these technical solutions will not overcome what is fundamentally a political problem. The author believes that comprehensive coverage will only come when the political environment changes.

Intermediate-Term and the Long Term

Lambrew, Jeanne, John D. Podesta, and Teresa L. Shaw. "Change in Challenging Times: A Plan for Extending and Improving Health Coverage." Health Affairs 23 (March 2005): 419–432. Are Americans neither politically capable nor morally committed to solving our health care problems? This is the question the authors ask, and ultimately argue against. They suggest that a health reform plan that balances practicality, fairness, and responsibility will work with American voters. They propose: a "value-added tax" (a national sales tax) would finance coverage for the uninsured; they would allow middle-income workers to use the federal employees health benefit plan (FEHBP); Medicaid would cover those workers and low-income Americans who currently have no insurance coverage.

Borger, Christine et al. "Health Spending Projections Through 2015: Changes on the Horizon." Health Affairs 22 (February 2006): W61-73.

Growth in national health spending is projected to slow down in 2005 to 7.4 percent, but still increase faster than overall economic growth, a trend that will continue over the next decade. During this time, we will see dramatic changes to our health care system, with the advent of prescription drug benefits in Medicare and the expanding numbers of Baby Boomers turning sixty-five. Even with private health insurance strategies to control costs, the authors estimate that health care spending will comprise twenty percent of the GDP by 2015.

Chernew, Michael E., Richard A. Hirth, and David M. Cutler. "Increased Spending on Health Care: How Much Can the United States Afford?" Health Affairs 22(4) (2003): 15–25. In this paper the authors develop a framework for thinking about affordability, concluding that if health expenditures increase at only two percent per year faster than personal income (a rate lower than historical trends), we can expect our standard of living to decline within the next few decades.

Blendon, Robert J., John M. Benson and Catherine M. DesRoches. "Americans' Views of the Uninsured: An Era for Hybrid Proposals." Health Affairs 27 (August, 2003): W3-405-414. Public opinion polls indicate that the issue of the uninsured remains important for Americans, and reports that in 2003, forty-three percent of Americans said they would support a "substantial" tax increase to achieve universal health care. The authors note that these findings need to be interpreted with care, as Americans tend to overstate what they are willing to pay, and that the public generally prefers rolling back tax cuts to address social needs rather than paying new taxes.

"Americans Favor Malpractice Reform and Drug Importation, But Rank Them Low on Health Priority List for the Congress and President." Kaiser Family Foundation, January 11, 2005. http://www.kff.org. According to this Kaiser Family Foundation and Harvard School of Public Health poll, almost two-thirds of U.S. adults say that lowering the cost of health insurance should be a top priority for the President and Congress. Stabilizing Medicare (fifty-eight percent) and reducing the number of uninsured (fifty-seven percent) followed as important priorities. Overall, health care issues ranked third in the survey, after the war in Iraq and behind economic issues.

INDEX

ABOUT THE AUTHORS

Arthur Garson Jr., MD, MPH, is Executive Vice President and Provost of the University of Virginia. From 2002–2007, he served as dean of the School of Medicine and of the University of Virginia. In 1999–2000, he served as president of the American College of Cardiology and forged principles for a reformed health care system now adopted by numerous physician groups. He is a member of the National Academies Institue of Medicine. In 2003, he was appointed by Health and Human Services Secretary Tommy Thompson to chair the National Advisory Council for the Agency for Healthcare Research and Quality, setting the first national five-year goals for quality. His expertise has been recognized by the Governors of North Carolina, Texas, and Virginia with appointments to chair state councils; he currently chairs the Virginia Health Reform Commission's Subcommittee on Healthcare Workforce and has recently co-chaired with the lt. governor a Subcommittee on Health Insurance Reform for small business. He recently developed and led drafting of federal legislation introduced in the U.S. Senate and House to provide federal grants for state innovation in health care coverage, quality, and cost. He continues to practice medicine, caring for children with heart disease.

Carolyn L. Engelhard, MPA, is assistant professor of medical education and a health policy analyst in the Department of Public Health Sciences at the University of Virginia School of Medicine, where she teaches health policy to undergraduates, graduate and medical students, and physicians in training. In addition, she directs the Master of Science program in clinical research in the Department of Public Health Sciences and provides technical and consultative services to state health and Medicaid agencies.